Evaluation *of* Health Care Quality *in* Advanced Practice Nursing

Joanne V. Hickey, PhD, APRN, ACNP-BC, FAAN, FCCM, is a Professor and holds the Patricia L. Starck/PARTNERS Professorship in Nursing at the University of Texas Health Science Center at Houston School of Nursing. She received a baccalaureate degree in nursing from Boston College, a master's of science degree in nursing from the University of Rhode Island, a master's of arts degree in counseling from Rhode Island College, a PhD degree from the University of Texas at Austin, and a post-master's certificate as a nurse practitioner from Duke University. She is certified by the American Nurses Credentialing Center as an acute care nurse practitioner, and the American Board of Neuroscience Nursing as a certified neuroscience registered nurse. She has served as an advanced practice nurse and consultant in the neurosciences and other acute/critical care areas at Massachusetts General Hospital, Duke University Medical Center, St. Lukes's Episcopal Hospital, and other facilities. She was the Scurlock Nurse Scholar at The Methodist's Hospital. Dr. Hickey has served as a consultant to clinical facilities nationally and internationally in evidence-based practice, advanced practice nursing, and doctor of nursing practice education. Dr. Hickey is the author of *The Clinical Practice of Neurological and Neurosurgical Nursing*, now in its sixth edition, and numerous articles on neuroscience topics and advanced practice issues. She is a frequent speaker at national and international conferences.

Christine A. Brosnan, DrPH, RN, is an Associate Professor of Nursing-Clinical at the University of Texas Health Science Center at Houston School of Nursing. She received a baccalaureate degree in nursing from Georgetown University, a master's of science degree in nursing from the University of Texas Medical Branch in Galveston, and a doctorate in public health from the University of Texas Health Science Center-Houston School of Public Health. The major area of study in her doctoral work was Health Services Organizations. Dr. Brosnan has collaborated in research studies on the cost and effectiveness of newborn screening and screening for hypertension and obesity in children. She has over thirty published articles, abstracts, chapters, proceedings, and letters, and has delivered numerous presentations on topics related to child health, screening, and economic evaluation. Her manuscript "Type 2 Diabetes in Children and Adolescents: An Emerging Disease" received the Excellence in Writing Award from the *Journal of Pediatric Health Care*.

Evaluation *of* Health Care Quality *in* Advanced Practice Nursing

Joanne V. Hickey, PhD, APRN, ACNP-BC, FAAN, FCCM

Christine A. Brosnan, DrPH, RN

SPRINGER PUBLISHING COMPANY
NEW YORK

Springer Publishing Company, LLC

11 West 42nd Street
New York, NY 10036
www.springerpub.com

Acquisitions Editor: Margaret Zuccarini
Composition: DiacriTech

ISBN: 978-0-8261-0766-4
E-book ISBN: 978-0-8261-0767-1

12 13 14 15 / 5 4 3 2 1

The author and the publisher of this Work have made every effort to use sources believed to be reliable to provide information that is accurate and compatible with the standards generally accepted at the time of publication. The author and publisher shall not be liable for any special, consequential, or exemplary damages resulting, in whole or in part, from the readers' use of, or reliance on, the information contained in this book. The publisher has no responsibility for the persistence or accuracy of URLs for external or third-party Internet Web sites referred to in this publication and does not guarantee that any content on such Web sites is, or will remain, accurate or appropriate.

Cataloging-in-Publication Data is available from the Library of Congress.

Special discounts on bulk quantities of our books are available to corporations, professional associations, pharmaceutical companies, health care organizations, and other qualifying groups.

If you are interested in a custom book, including chapters from more than one of our titles, we can provide that service as well.

For details, please contact:
Special Sales Department, Springer Publishing Company, LLC
11 West 42nd Street, 15th Floor, New York, NY 10036-8002s
Phone: 877-687-7476 or 212-431-4370; Fax: 212-941-7842
Email: sales@springerpub.com

Printed in the United States of America by Bang Printing

We dedicate this book to ...

- *Pioneers and thought leaders* ... the pioneers in the field of evaluation, including Florence Nightingale, Ernest Codman, Avedis Donabedian, and Lu Ann Aday, who have elevated evaluation to a science-based process; and the thought leaders who are demanding that a solid evaluation must be an integral part in all health care endeavors.
- *Students and colleague (current and future)* ... and particularly advanced practice nurses who have an unprecedented opportunity to impact new models of health care quality that will influence health policy for an ultimate transformation of the health care system.
- *Our contributing authors* ... recognized experts in their disciplines, these leaders are much sought after for their expertise in practice, education, research, and consultation. Our request to share their knowledge through writing was met with gracious acceptance and production of excellent manuscripts. Their passion for quality health care and especially the role of evaluation in achieving quality health care is the heart and soul of this book.
- *Our husbands* ... who supported our passion for creating this book even though it took considerable time away from other home- and family-based activities. Jim Hickey and Pat Brosnan served as in-house editors and wise listeners and counsels as we grappled with the best ways to organize ideas and find the right words to illuminate the work of evaluation.

Contents

Contributors

Christine A. Brosnan, DrPH, RN
Associate Professor of Nursing-Clinical at the University of Texas Health
Science Center at Houston School of Nursing, Houston, Texas

Maureen Disbot, MS, RN, CCRN
Vice President, Quality Operations, The Methodist Hospital, Houston, Texas

Deanna E. Grimes, DrPH, RN, FAAN
Professor, Division Head, Community Health Nursing, Director, MSN/MPH
Program with University of Texas School of Public Health, University of
Texas Health Science Center at Houston School of Nursing, Houston, Texas

Richard M. Grimes, PhD, MBA
Adjunct Professor, University of Texas Health Science Center at Houston
Medical School, Houston, Texas

Joanne V. Hickey, PhD, APRN, ACNP-BC, FAAN, FCCM
Professor, University of Texas Health Science Center at Houston
School of Nursing, Houston, Texas

Sharon McLane, PhD, MBA, RN-BC
Director of Clinical Transformation, Lakeland Regional Medical Center,
Lakeland, Florida

Ronda G. Hughes, PhD, MHS, RN, FAAN
Associate Professor, Marquette University, College of Nursing, Milwaukee,
Wisconsin

Ann Scanlon-McGinity, PhD, RN, FAAN
Chief Nurse Executive, Senior Vice President, Operations, The Methodist
Hospital, Houston, Texas

J. Michael Swint, PhD
Professor of Health Economics, George McMillan Fleming Professor,
Director, Division of Management, Policy, and Community Health,
University of Texas Health Science Center at Houston School of Public
Health, Houston, Texas

Nancy F. Weller, DrPh, MPH, MS, RN
Assistant Professor of Nursing, Clinical, University of Texas Health Science
Center at Houston School of Nursing, Houston, Texas

Preface

Evaluation is not a new concept to nurses. It is most often associated with a component of the nursing process designed to evaluate the outcomes of health care for an individual patient. Competency in evaluation of patient outcomes is an expectation of all professional nurses. What is new is the expectation of high level competency for advanced practice nurses (APNs) in evaluating health care, including health professional groups, patient populations, organizations, systems, programs, health informatics, practice guidelines/protocols, health policy, and other health-related entities from a systematic and comprehensive evaluation perspective. The bar for evaluation has been raised for APNs. Along with the higher expectations comes a new opportunity to influence high level decision making in health care.

Recognizing the need for APNs to be prepared in evaluation beyond individual patients, we conducted a search to identify textbooks and other resources that would be helpful for APNs to conduct their work. Surprisingly, little was found beyond case studies and general principles, although there were several books on program evaluation. Although helpful, these resources did not address the full scope of evaluation required in advanced practice nursing. No one comprehensive text was found that addressed the most common foci of evaluation by APNs. With this background we began the planning of this text guided by input from our colleagues, students, and practicing APNs. Our esteemed colleagues graciously agreed to share their expertise through the written word.

The intended audiences are students enrolled in advanced practice nursing programs, practicing APNs both at the master's, and doctoral levels, nurse administrators, directors of quality improvement, faculty teaching evaluators, and others interested in evaluation of health care from a practice and clinical perspective. In selecting content, it was our intention to provide an overview of the state of the science of evaluation and what is known about evaluation and its application to common practice issues in which ANPs will lead or participate. As we reviewed the literature it became clear that evaluation as applied to health care is underdeveloped and evolving. It is a non-linear and messy process; there is no one right way to conduct an evaluation. The form of an evaluation is based on its intended purpose and use. The clear and urgent message is that all aspects of health care entities must be evaluated systematically for effectiveness and to guide and inform decision making. APNs can contribute to developing the science, processes, and uses of evaluation in health care. Although the consensus is in agreement with a national call to action, the processes and timelines for evaluation are poorly established. The intent of this book is to lay a foundation for APNs to assume their important role in evaluation.

Section I addresses the underpinning of evaluation. Chapter 1 elaborates on the role of APNs in evaluation. Through a brief history, overview, mandate, and other aspects of high level evaluation, the APN is brought to the table of evaluation. Chapter 2 addresses the nature of evidence, the basic building block of evaluation, and provides a critical review of characteristics, sources, and quality of evidence as it applies to rigorous evaluation. The conceptual foundations for evaluation are discussed in Chapter 3. A number of frameworks are described to provide the reader with different models for addressing evaluation. The national imperative for cost effectiveness is addressed in Chapter 4 through an overview of economic evaluation.

Evaluation of organizations, systems, and standards for practice is the focus of Section II. Chapter 5 examines evaluation of organizations and systems, while Chapter 6 addresses health care informatics and patient care technology within health care. With the redesign of health care delivery, organizations and systems are being restructured and redesigned to be more responsive to patient-family centered care models. An integral part of health care is health informatics, and patient care technology integration and evaluation. The current national trend toward electronic medical records is creating challenges because of the far reaching impact on organizations, systems, and individual patients.

Section III addresses the evaluation of populations and health care teams. From a lens of populations, Chapter 8 addresses characteristics, risk factors, determinants, and the evaluation of population health. Chapter 9 covers the emphasis on interdisciplinary collaborative health teams as the foundation for quality and safety outcomes.

The final section, Section IV, is devoted to health policy and the future of health care evaluation. Chapter 10 discusses the important step of translating outcomes from evaluation into health policy. The chapter encourages APNs to seek opportunities for advocacy and leadership in developing new policies or revision of current health care policy. Chapter 11 examines challenges and trends for the future including the increased demand for comprehensive high level evaluation by APNs. In addition, the chapter addresses recommendations about initial and ongoing competency in evaluation by APNs.

Some of the unique features of the book are key definitions of terms, multiple examples to illustrate a point, case studies to provide examples of comprehensive evaluations with clinical applications and recommended resources for perusal and reference. As educators and practitioners, we were keenly aware of the multiple definitions of key terms. Unless evaluators and users of evaluations are clear about terminology, confusion and misunderstandings will abound leading to underutilized or misdirected evaluations. The examples in the book come from a variety of practice settings and foci to provide the reader with an appreciation of the multiple uses of evaluation. This is also true of the case studies, which provide a more comprehensive overview of the evaluation process, outcomes, and uses. Readers may wish to explore other resources to augment their understanding and broaden their perspective of aspects of evaluation. Selected resources are thus provided for these purposes.

Our sincere hope is that this book will meet our primary aim of providing a useful and helpful resource to assist APNs in assuming responsibility and accountability for competency in the conduct of high level evaluation that will inform decision making for those engaged in health care delivery and practice. Competency in high quality evaluation positions APNs to influence health care decisions and health policy. It speaks loudly to the recommendation outlined in *The Future of Nursing: Leading Change, Advancing Health* (Institute of Medicine, 2011) that nurses should be full partners with other health professionals in redesigning health care.

Acknowledgments

We are indebted to many wonderful people who helped to make this book possible. We especially wish to acknowledge Dr. LuAnn Aday for her helpful review of the conceptual models of evaluation discussed in Chapter 3.

ONE

Evaluation in Advanced Practice Nursing

Joanne V. Hickey and Christine A. Brosnan

"What we call the beginning is often the end.
And to make an end is to make a beginning.
The end is where we start from."

T. S. Eliot

INTRODUCTION

Within the current national imperatives for health care quality and safety, the mandate for evaluation of care has never been more vital to meeting societal needs. Quality care is safe care, and safe care is a hallmark of quality. Evaluating the quality of care delivered to clients/patients is a necessity that emerges from the social contract between health professionals and society. Implicit in this social contract is the accountability of all health professionals to their clients/patients for the quality and safety of the services they render and for the expectation of care with predictable outcomes (Sidani & Braden, 1998).

This book examines the theory and practice of evaluation in advanced practice nursing. All professional registered nurses evaluate care provided to individual patients as part of the nursing process. The American Nurses Association (ANA, 2010, p. 63) defines evaluation as the process of determining the progress toward attainment of expected outcomes including the effectiveness of care. *Bloom's Taxonomy of the Cognitive Domain* (B. Bloom, Enlerhart, Furst, Hill, & Krathwohl, 1956) is a time-honored hierarchy of cognitive abilities arranged from the least complex to the most complex. The original taxonomy was arranged in the following order: knowledge, comprehension, application, analysis, synthesis, and evaluation. Each of the preceding levels is foundational for the subsequent level, and evaluation is at the highest level of complexity in the cognitive domain. Other authors have suggested that synthesis and evaluation are at the same level of difficulty, but use different cognitive processes (Anderson & Krathwohl, 2001). Regardless of these differences of opinion, it is clear that evaluation is a high-level cognitive activity that is complex in nature. Benner, Hughes, and Sutphen (2008) note that high order critical thinking and clinical reasoning are required for high quality clinical practice.

The ANA's definition of evaluation is a *discipline-focused* definition of the patient's responses to interventions and specific outcomes, as well as the care provided by the nurse. The advanced practice nurse (APN) must move beyond the single patient/client- and discipline-specific focus to also address evaluation at a population, organizational, systems, and provider level. With this perspective, the APN expands the depth and scope of evaluation to include the theoretical and scientific approaches utilized by behavioral, social, and organizational scientists to evaluate more complex multidisciplinary questions. The theoretical foundation of evaluation is grounded in science and the rigorous methodologies used to conduct systematic evaluations of phenomena of interest to those engaged in the delivery and utilization of health care services. In order for any evaluation to have credibility, it must be based on the best practices of evaluation science and methodologies considered to be valid and reliable by industry standards.

The APN must engage in evaluation at this level of expertise to be viewed as a credible health professional by health and other professionals, administrators, decision makers, and leaders who have expertise in evaluation science and methodologies. The results of these evaluations are used to inform decision makers who will affect health care delivery and the health care systems. The focus of an evaluation can be broad and comprehensive and may include quality indicators, clinical outcomes, and the risks–benefits of health care for a population, an organization, or a system. Table 1.1 provides examples of the scope of evaluation possibilities in which APNs might engage. The contributions of APNs is integral to achieving a high quality health care system for the nation, and thus APNs must develop the competencies to engage in high level evaluations processes both independently and as a member of a multidisciplinary team. Only then will the full potential of the APN to achieve high quality and safe outcomes be realized. It is, therefore, the primary purpose of this book to assist APNs to understand evaluation as an integral component of advanced practice and the theoretical and scientific underpinnings of evaluation in the health care system.

The differentiation of microsystem, mesosystem, and macrosystem influences evaluation. A *microsystem* refers to the small, functional frontline units that provide most health care to most people (Nelson et al., 2007, p. 3). A *mesosystem* is a larger unit in which midlevel leaders are responsible for large clinical programs, clinical support services, and administrative services

TABLE 1.1

Examples of Evaluations in Advanced Practice Nursing

Focus	Description	Example
Patient/client or groups/populations		
Groups of patients/ clients	A group may be defined as a group of patients who have in common a provider(s), disease, or receive care in a particular setting. Focus of patient-centered evaluation is usually directed at response to care and health outcomes.	In a diabetic group within a practice, how the patients/clients' outcomes compare to national, evidence-based guidelines such as targeted HgbA1c, weight, and blood pressure levels.
Populations	Refers to a set of persons having a common personal or environmental characteristic. The common characteristic may be anything that influences health such as age, diagnosis, level of disability, etc. (Maurer & Smith, 2004).	The outcomes of patients with ischemic stroke in a multi-facility health care system as compared with national guidelines. Patient satisfaction with care and the encounter with the health care system.
Organization		
Models of care	A conceptual model or diagram that broadly defines the way health services are delivered.	The effectiveness of models of practice such as interprofessional teams or solo practice in achieving decreased length of stay.
Evidence-based practice	The integration of best research evidence, clinical research, and patient values in making decisions about the care of individual patients (IOM, 2003).	The adherence to evidence-based guidelines for myocardial infarction as the patient moved from one unit to another along the continuum of care.
Quality improvement	A formal approach to the analysis of performance and systematic efforts to improve it through a planned program within an organization.	Integration of health care technology and information systems into point of service care for a particular diagnosis or condition.

(continued)

TABLE 1.1

Examples of Evaluations in Advanced Practice Nursing (*continued*)

Focus	Description	Example
Systems		
Cost effective- ness analysis (CEA)	A comparative evaluation of two or more interventions in which costs are calculated in dollars (or the local currency) and end-points are calculated in health related units (Drummond, Sculpher, Torrance, O'Briend, & Stoddart, 2005).	Assists health profess- ionals in making deci- sions about equipment purchases or establish- ing new programs or services.
Responsiveness to community needs	The ability of a person, unit, or organization to address the expressed needs of a community. The community is usually described as external to the health care organization or system and may be people living in the same area as the facility, a facility such as a housing project, or an ethnic group with ties to the health care facility.	Programs are developed based on expressed needs of the community of interest through a partnership with that community so that the community partners are stakeholders in the program. Examples of such programs are starting a Saturday clinic for immunization at the local school, a prenatal clinic for high-risk mothers in a community with a high incidence of premature deliveries, or a hypertension clinic at a local industrial plant for workers.

(Nelson et al., 2007, p. 205). It is the layer between the microsystem and the macrosystem, and is often the interface between the two. A *macrosystem* refers to broader, overarching sectors such as organizations or systems. Its leaders are responsible for organization-wide performance (Nelson et al., 2007, p. 205). Depending upon the purpose, the evaluation can focus on a single level (e.g., microsystem, mesosystem, or macrosystem), or can include all three levels. At the micro level, the emphasis is on evaluating the quality of a particular inter- vention or program, and often involves examining the effectiveness in achiev- ing expected outcomes (Sidani & Braden, 1998). An evaluation addressing a problem at the mesosystem level may focus on a division, such as surgical services, in which multiple units that provide clinical care to surgical patients are included. An example of a possible evaluation focus might be policies and procedures for the clinical service. At the macro level, the emphasis shifts to a broad and comprehensive focus in which evaluation of the quality of programs or initiatives at the organization or systems level is addressed. For example, an evaluation might investigate the organizational policies on drug reconciliation as patients move from one unit to another.

EVALUATION AND RELATED TERMS AND CONCEPTS

There are many definitions of evaluation, and some are reflective of a specific type of evaluation. Table 1.2 includes terms commonly used in evaluation. A generic definition of evaluation is: A process that requires judgments to be made about the extent to which something satisfies a criterion or criteria; another definition is "The systematic application of scientific and statistical procedures for measuring program conceptualization, design, implementation, and utility; making comparisons based on these measurement; and the use of the resulting information to optimize program outcome" (Centers for Disease Control and Prevention [CDC], 1999). This is a broader definition than the ANA definition given earlier and focuses mainly on programs. Other related terms and concepts often used have some commonalities as

TABLE 1.2
Definitions of Frequently Used Terms in Evaluation of Health Care

Term	Definitions
Accountability	The obligation to demonstrate and take responsibility for performance in light of agreed expectations.
Analysis	An investigation of the component parts of a whole and their relationships in making up the whole; the process of breaking a complex topic or substance into smaller parts to gain a better understanding of it.
Assessment	The classification of someone or something with respect to its worth.
Benchmarking	The process of comparing one's processes and performance metrics to industry bests and/or best practices from other industries.
Best practices	The most up-to-date patient care interventions, which result in the best patient outcomes and minimal patient risk of complications or death (RWJF, 2011).

(continued)

TABLE 1.2

Definitions of Frequently Used Terms in Evaluation of Health Care (*continued*)

Term	Definitions
Criterion	A standard on which a judgment or decision may be based. "an attribute of structure, process, or outcome that is used to draw an inference about quality" (Donabedian, 2003, p. 60).
Critique	A critical review of an object, process, literature, or performance; a critical examination or estimate of a thing or situation with the view to determine its nature and limitations or its conformity to standards or criteria.
Effectiveness	The degree to which goals and objectives are successfully met. Refers to a change in health status resulting from an intervention provided under usual conditions (Donabedian, 2003, p. 4).
Efficacy	The degree to which an intervention can be effective under optimum implementation conditions.
Evaluation	The process of determining the progress toward attainment of expected outcomes including the effectiveness of care (ANA, 2010, p. 63).
	"The systematic application of scientific and statistical procedures for measuring program conceptualization, design, implementation, and utility; making comparisons based on these measurement; and the use of the resulting information to optimize program outcome" (CDC, 1999).
Formative evaluation	An appraisal occurring during the implementation of an intervention (such as a program or patient interaction).
Indicators	A quantitative or qualitative variable that provides simple and reliable means to measure achievement, monitor performance, or to reflect changes.
Monitor	The process of comparing one's business processes and performance metrics to industry bests and/or best practices from other industries.
Quality	Medical quality is the degree to which health care systems, services, and supplies for individuals and populations increase the likelihood for positive health outcomes and are consistent with current professional knowledge (IOM, 1990).
Quality assurance	A program for the systematic monitoring and evaluation of the various aspects of a project, service, or facility to ensure that standards of quality are being met. "All actions taken to establish, protect, promote, and improve the quality of health care" (Donabedian, 2003a, p. xxiv).

(*continued*)

TABLE 1.2 (*continued*)

Term	Definitions
Quality of care	A measure of the ability of the provider, health care facility, or health plan to provide services for individuals and populations that increase the likelihood of desired health outcomes and are consistent with current professional knowledge (RWJF, 2011).
Quality improvement	Initiatives with a goal to improve the processes or outcomes of the care being delivered.
	Clinical quality improvement is an interdisciplinary process designed to raise the standards of the delivery of preventive, diagnostic, therapeutic, and rehabilitative measures in order to maintain, restore, or improve health outcomes of individuals and populations (IOM, 1990).
Standard	Authoritative statement established and promulgated by credible sources such as the profession by which the quality of practice, service, or education can be judged (ANA, 2004).
Summative evaluation	An appraisal that occurs at the end of an intervention or program.
Synthesis	The composition or combination of parts or elements so as to form a whole; the combining or often diverse conceptions into a coherent whole.
Transparency	"The process of collecting and reporting health care cost, performance, and quality data in a format that can be accessed by the public and is intended to improve the delivery of service and ultimately improve the health care system" (RWJF, 2011).
	Ensuring openness in the delivery of serves and practices with particular emphasis on valid, reliable, accessible, timely, and meaningful data that are readily available to stakeholders including the public.

well as differences with evaluation that include program evaluation, quality assurance, quality improvement, and outcomes research.

Program evaluation, as viewed from a public health lens, is defined as "an essential organizational practice in public health using a systematic approach to improve and account for public health actions" (CDC, 1999). *Quality improvement* is a process of assessment conducted about a patient's care or an organizational or systems problem for the purpose of improving processes or outcomes. *Quality assurance* is defined as "all actions taken to establish, protect, promote, and improve the quality of health care" (Donabedian, 2003b,

p. xxiii). Quality assurance is the older term and still used in the literature, although quality improvement is the term seen more frequently.

A BRIEF HISTORY OF HEALTH CARE EVALUATION

Individuals change history, and the modern history of health care evaluation was particularly influenced by three visionaries: Florence Nightingale, Ernest Codman, and Avedis Donabedian. Each brought to health care the idea that interventions should be more than worthy efforts and should produce real benefit to patients. It is said that Florence Nightingale not only took care of patients, she also counted them. Born in 1820, she was drawn to mathematics, nursing, and public health, none of which was considered a desirable career for a wealthy woman living in 19th century England (Spiegelhalter, 1999). As a professional nurse, she had the vision to integrate her keen observational skills with her knowledge of statistics and public health to improve patient care. Nightingale is a recognized pioneer in the evaluation of health care outcomes because she clearly understood the goal of care. She said, "In dwelling upon the vital importance of *sound* observation, it must never be lost sight of what observation is for. It is not for the sake of piling up miscellaneous information or curious facts, but for the sake of saving life and increasing health and comfort" (Nightingale, 1859, p. 70).

Ernest Codman was a man who lived before his time. He was born in 1869 and educated at Harvard Medical School. He accepted a position at Massachusetts General Hospital soon after graduation and seemed to be following the path of a successful physician of his day (Archives of the American College of Surgeons; Donabedian, 1989). But he began to wonder if medical interventions actually improved patient health and soon focused on the idea of measuring end results. He left Massachusetts General Hospital to found his own hospital in which he put his theories about evaluation into practice. In 1924, he described his concept of end result: "It is that every hospital should tract each patient with the object of ascertaining whether the maximum benefit has been obtained and to find out if not, why not" (Codman, 2009, pp. 2766–2770).

Dr. Codman kept cards on each of his patients. On each card he would write how he had treated a patient and whether his treatment helped or hurt. He had patients with similar conditions placed on the same wards and suggested they should be under the care of a physician with specialized knowledge about the condition. He collected patient information during a hospital stay and analyzed it to determine the success or failure of medical care. He encouraged his colleagues to do as he did, but very few shared his enthusiasm or curiosity. The more he exhorted members of the medical community to examine the results of their interventions, the more they distanced themselves from him. The preoccupation with using patient outcomes to learn about improving care changed the course of his life and resulted in some success. He integrated his ideas into projects and published works, which received acclaim during his lifetime. But he was never able to convince his colleagues that evaluating medical care would lead to improved patient health (Donabedian, 1989).

Avedis Donabedian developed a model for health care evaluation that is still widely used today. Born in 1919, Dr. Donabedian spent a major portion of his professional career teaching and writing at the University of Michigan (Sunōl, 2000). He discerned that health care outcomes could not be measured in isolation (Mulley, 1989); rather, they must be viewed within the context of the quality of care (Donabedian, 1980). He understood that methodologies must differ based on the perspective of the evaluation. That is, the methods used to evaluate the quality of care to an individual patient are different than the methods used to evaluate system or population outcomes (Donabedian, 1980).

Donabedian (1980) defined quality as "a judgment concerning the process of care, based on the extent to which care contributes to valued outcomes" and outlined indicators of *structure, process*, and *outcome* as pathways to evaluating quality of care. He described structure as "the relatively stable characteristics of the providers of care, of the tools and resources they have at their disposal and of the physical and organizational settings in which they work" (Donabedian, 1980). He described process as "a set of activities that go on within and between practitioners and patients," and outcomes as "a change in a patient's current and future health status that can be attributed to antecedent health care" (Donabedian, 1980).

Each of these leaders had an unswerving dedication to improving patient health. They had the clarity of vision to see the link between practitioner-patient interactions and health status, and the perseverance to continue their work regardless of the obstacles. Their influence continues to impact health care evaluation and quality improvement science today.

WHY IS EVALUATION SOMETIMES NEGLECTED?

There are a number of reasons why so many resources are spent on developing new interventions and programs while comparatively little time is spent on evaluating them. First, the concept of evaluation itself is threatening. Most practitioners follow care protocols they believe will produce good outcomes if applied competently. Evaluating care can be seen as questioning the practitioners' personal dedication, knowledge and skills. Second, the available evidence may be insufficient to determine if a treatment or program is really effective. Practitioners may follow protocols and still have poor outcomes because they are doing the wrong thing right. The standard of care is only as good as the evidence supporting it.

Third, evaluation is difficult and complex (Mulley, 1989). For example, in the intensive care unit, practitioners must adjust for patient demographic characteristics and prior health status before measuring patient outcomes.

Age, gender, socioeconomic status, and severity of illness all factor into developing a case mix. Feasibility must also be considered. Tracking of indicators of care over a long period of time may be essential to determine if a program benefits a population but this may be seen as too costly and impractical.

Fourth, technology keeps changing. Practitioners may find themselves in the middle of evaluating a program when new information or a new technique makes the program obsolete. Finally, innovation is exciting and often brings funding and acclaim to a system or institution. Evaluation can seem a necessary but tedious process that diverts resources and time away from patient care (M. Bloom, Fischer, & Orme, 1999).

The case of hormone replacement therapy (HRT) is a good example of the complexities inherent in evaluating interventions. Practitioners had long recognized that HRT provided relief to menopausal women from the effects of vasomotor symptoms such as hot flashes and night sweats. During the 1990s reviews of mainly observational studies indicated HRT had additional benefits including a decrease in both cardiovascular disease and hip fractures (Barrett-Connor, Grady, & Stefanick, 2005). HRT treatment for menopausal women became the standard of care and prescriptions soared, climbing to 91 million in 2001 (Hersch, Stefanick, & Stafford, 2004). Practitioners followed protocols and diligently recommended HRT to their patients because they thought it was the right thing to do. Patients learned about the importance of hormone therapy from newspaper articles, the Internet, and TV and were glad to take a pill that might prevent serious and debilitating disorders. A few practitioners may have observed adverse events among their patients, but probably not enough to be alarming. An individual practitioner lacked the sample size to detect a significant increase in morbidity or mortality.

Then findings from the Women's Health Initiative Estrogen Plus Progestin Trial (WHI-EPT) and the Heart and Estrogen/Progestin Replacement Study (HERS) were released (Hulley et al., 1998; Rossouw et al., 2002). These studies were randomized controlled trials and involved thousands of women. Depending upon the kind of hormone medication prescribed, results indicated that women had an increased risk for certain cardiovascular diseases and cancers. The number of prescriptions plummeted as the standard of care changed and practitioners became more cautious in their treatment. This case illustrates that an individual practitioner frequently lacks the resources and expertise to evaluate a new and widely accepted intervention that becomes the standard of care. It is also an example of practitioners unwittingly doing the wrong thing right.

AN OVERVIEW OF HEALTH CARE EVALUATION

Health care evaluation may be described as a systematic and objective determination of the structure, process, and outcomes of care. The goal of evaluation is to provide the practitioner with the information needed to make decisions about future actions. Evaluation is most often a collaborative process because the very nature of health care is collaborative. The APN works with other professional practitioners in providing patient care and, similarly, the APN usually collaborates with other health professionals to arrive at a judgment about the benefits, risks, and cost of care.

The APN is one member of a team comprising professionals who have the skill and knowledge to contribute their expertise to the endeavor. Depending upon the purpose, perspective, depth, and scope of the evaluation, team members may include stakeholders, economists, administrators, politicians, patients, and other health care professionals. The team leader should be selected based on unique expertise required for the specific project and team members should be assigned tasks based on their unique skills. During the planning phase of the study, the team leader should have frequent discussions with the administrator or sponsor requesting the evaluation. This is to ensure that the goal and purpose of the study are clearly understood, that methods are appropriate to the setting, and that adequate financial and structural support will be provided.

The first step in developing an evaluation plan is to discuss the purpose of the evaluation (Table 1.3). The purpose may be to examine only one approach (for example, the outcome of care) or to examine all three approaches to quality assurance (the structure, process, and outcome of care). An outcome evaluation may focus on the *effectiveness* of an intervention, program, or policy. *Effectiveness* refers to a change in health status resulting from an intervention provided under usual conditions. Effectiveness differs from *efficacy*, a term frequently used to describe a change in health status resulting from an intervention provided under controlled conditions (Brook & Lohr, 1985; Donabedian, 2003a).

The team may choose to conduct a formative evaluation or a summative evaluation. *Formative evaluation* refers to an appraisal occurring during the implementation of a program in which the results are used to revise and improve the rest of the program. *Summative evaluation* refers to an appraisal that occurs at the end of a program in which the results are used

TABLE 1.3
Steps in the Evaluation Process

Decide on the purpose of the study.
Determine the perspective of the study.
Select a conceptual model.
Choose an appropriate and feasible study design. Determine methodology.
Conduct the study.
Submit results in a written report and/or oral presentation.

to determine the benefit and future use of the program. Formative is often used interchangeably with process evaluation, and summative evaluation is used interchangeably with outcome. They do not always mean the same thing (Fitzpatrick, Sanders, & Worthen, 2004).

For example, as part of a hospital program to prevent nosocomial infections, a practitioner conducts a process evaluation to determine if the correct protocol for hand washing is being used by the staff. The evaluation is formative if data about hand washing methods are collected during the course of the evaluation and used to make adjustments to the current hand washing protocol. The evaluation is summative if data about hand washing methods are collected at the end of the evaluation and used to modify future programs to prevent nosocomial infections. In each case the evaluation focused on a process of care (hand washing) but differed on how the results were used.

Second, the team determines the evaluation's perspective. Will the evaluation be viewed from the perspective of an individual, an organization (such as a hospital or clinic facility), or society (such as a city, state, or country). Methods vary depending upon the perspective of the study. Third, the team selects a compatible conceptual model. The conceptual model provides the framework from which evaluation activities flow. Donabedian's model has been briefly described, and will be further discussed in the next chapter along with other evaluation models. Fourth, the team chooses an appropriate evaluation design and methods. There are several alternatives from which to choose depending upon the type of evaluation and the resources available. One alternative is to identify criteria of interest, collect data, and compare the findings to a standard that may be internally developed or externally required by an accrediting body or government agency. A *criterion* refers to characteristics used to appraise the quality of care. A *standard* refers to a measurable reference point that is used for comparison. Generally, criteria are expressed in relation to standards (Donabedian, 2003a; Fitzpatrick et al., 2004). For example, if an evaluation is focused on diabetes mellitus management, an appropriate criterion could be the level of HgbA1c. The standard might be "95% of clinic patients will maintain a HgbA1c <7%."

The team decides on the methods they will use to assess and analyze data collected. In this context, *assessment* is part of the methodology and refers to the collection of data. *Monitoring* refers to the periodically scheduled collection of data. Monitoring may be used to detect trends and to determine compliance with guidelines and protocols (Donabedian, 2003a; Fitzpatrick et al., 2004). The team selects the type of data to be collected, the most suitable sources of data, the instruments that will be used to collect data, the time period for data collection, and the personnel responsible for gathering the data. In the preceding example, evaluators could, over the course of a year, retrospectively monitor the medical records of a sample of patients with diabetes.

Analysis refers to the procedures and calculations used to describe or make inferences about the data collected. Depending upon the perspective and scope of the appraisal, analysis may be as simple as comparing the results of the evaluation to a standard. For example, data obtained from a retrospective medical record review might be analyzed and the mean value for each patient calculated. The percent of patients who maintained a HgbA1c <7% would then be determined and the results compared to the standard of 95%. In contrast, analysis of complex designs may require application of sophisticated statistical techniques.

Fifth, the team conducts the evaluation. The number of personnel and resources needed to implement the study depends upon the complexity and scope of the evaluation. A plan that is clear and understood by everyone involved will greatly increase the chance of success. Sixth, the team submits a report that clearly describes the results, including strengths and weaknesses of the evaluation, conclusions, and implications. Team members review the findings and discuss their recommendations with the administrator or sponsor requesting the evaluation.

THE DIFFERENCES BETWEEN RESEARCH EVALUATION AND NON-RESEARCH EVALUATION

Evaluation activities that are categorized as research and activities categorized as non-research share similarities. All evaluations are systematic and objective; they flow from a conceptual framework, make comparisons, and draw conclusions. However, there are characteristics that are more likely to be associated with one or the other (Table 1.4). Quality improvement and program evaluation are generally assumed to fall into the category of non-research (CDC, 1999; Morris & Dracup, 2007; Newhouse, 2007). Outcomes research and health service research are generally assumed to fall into the category of research. It is important to understand the distinction between research and non-research evaluation to ensure that evaluation activities are conducted in an ethical and legal manner.

TABLE 1.4
A Comparison of Non-Research Evaluation and Research Evaluation

Component	Non-Research Evaluation	Research Evaluation
Purpose	Improves current health care practice or health policy.	May or may not impact health care practice or health policy.
	Evaluates standard practice or clinical guidelines.	Generates new knowledge including the effectiveness of new interventions.

(continued)

TABLE 1.4

A Comparison of Non-Research Evaluation and Research Evaluation (*continued*)

Component	Non-Research Evaluation	Research Evaluation
Study design and methods	Design is normally less rigorous than research. Structure-process-outcome criteria may be monitored over time. Frequently reviews medical records. Often includes comparisons to an internal or external standard.	Often includes controls or randomization. Clinical trials and observational studies are more frequently used. Data are obtained from a wide variety of sources. Describes findings in one group or compares groups.
Patient risk	Minimal or none.	Patient risk is usually increased.
Implementation	Leadership depends upon the purpose and the individual expertise of team members.	Principal investigator of the research team writes the grant proposal and organizes the process.
Submit results	Results are not usually generalizable. Results are submitted to the individual or group sponsoring the evaluation. Results may or may not be published. Findings are used internally to improve a specific program or practice.	There is an expectation that results are generalizable. Process includes submitting the results for publication. Findings become part of a growing body of science.

The purpose of research evaluation is to generate new knowledge that may or may not directly improve current health practice or patient health status (M. Bloom et al., 1999). Whether a non-research evaluation examines an intervention, a program, or a policy, the purpose is to directly improve current health practice and patient status. The evaluator is monitoring an accepted and standard practice. The purpose is *not* to generate new knowledge. Research as described in 45CFR 46.102(d) is "a systematic investigation, including research development, testing and evaluation designed to develop or contribute to generalizable knowledge" (CDC, 1999; U.S. Department of Health & Human Services [USDHHS], 2009).

Types of research designs and methods may overlap in evaluation but research evaluation is likely to apply more rigorous designs including controls and randomization (McNett & Lawry, 2009). Randomized controlled trials and observational designs are frequently used in research and data are obtained from a wide variety of sources. Non-research evaluation is more likely than research to monitor structure-process-outcome criteria through medical record review. Findings are compared to an internal or external standard rather than to a similar group of patients.

A key difference between non-research and research evaluation involves patient risk (Reinhardt & Ray, 2003). Research places patients at greater risk than they would be under standard clinical protocols. The testing of a new intervention, a rigorous design, and the desire to generalize findings require the collection of data that are not needed for standard health practice (Casarett, Karlawish, & Sugarman, 2000). Prior to beginning a study that involves human subjects, researchers must submit a study proposal to the Institutional Review Board (IRB) of a hospital or agency. The Board may decide that the study is exempt from review or that a review is needed before approval can be given allowing investigators to proceed. Non-research evaluation is exempt from IRB review (USDHHS, 2009).

In research studies, the principal investigator selects an area of interest, writes a proposal for funding, and assumes leadership of the project (Fitzpatrick et al., 2004, p. 6). Non-research evaluations are frequently made at the request of administrators, policy makers, politicians, or stakeholders. The team member with the greatest expertise in the area assumes leadership. The APN may be a leader in an evaluation focused on nursing care and a team member in an evaluation focused on respiratory care.

There is an expectation in research that the findings are generalizable and that results will be published in order to expand scientific knowledge (CDC, 1999). Results from a non-research evaluation are not necessarily generalizable and are usually not published. Instead, a report is presented internally to the administrators who requested the study. Administrators then decide whether or not to use the recommendation to change health care practice, revise an existing program, or modify policy.

Distinguishing research evaluation from non-research evaluation can be difficult. Experts in the field continue to debate the attributes of each category (Miller & Emanuel, 2008). Saying that an evaluation is being done for the purpose of quality improvement or program evaluation does not eliminate the possibility that the study meets the definition of research and that the proposal must be submitted to an IRB. One way to address this concern is to appoint an administrator with experience in evaluation who reviews all evaluation studies before implementation and collaborates with IRB members to confirm that correct procedures are followed (McNett & Lawry, 2009).

THE RELATIONSHIP OF POLICY AND ADVANCED PRACTICE

A policy refers to a plan of action that incorporates goals and procedures (Guralnik, 1979; Merriam-Webster Dictionary). Health care policies may be organizational or societal. They evolve from scientific evidence, cultural values, and political influence. The development of rules for patient visitation provides an example of the factors impacting policy decisions. Nightingale (1859), among others, discussed the benefits and harms of visitors to patient well-being. There has been a longstanding debate among health care professionals about who should be allowed to visit and the timing of visits in hospital units, particularly in specialty care units. Concerns included increased risk of infection, lack of time available to interact with families, and confidentiality issues (DeLeskey, 2009; Frazier, Frazier, & Warren, 2010; Kamerling, Lawler, Lynch, & Schwartz, 2008; Powazek, Goff, Schyving, & Paulson, 1978).

Changing cultural mores affected this debate as patients along with their families and friends became vocal about having input into the decision-making process. Policies changed as evidence indicated the benefit to patients when those close to them are allowed to visit (Walls, 2009). At the micro level, individual hospitals developed policies that encouraged family visits. Kamerling et al. (2008) described a quality improvement program designed to increase visitation through a multidisciplinary collaboration of family and health care professionals, through staff education, and through increased administrative support. Over a 3-year period, visitation increased from 44% to 90%. At the macro level, on April 15, 2010, President Barak Obama (2010) signed a memo directing the Secretary of Health and Human Services "to ensure that hospitals that participate in Medicare or Medicaid respect the rights of patients to designate visitors".

Policy formulation and implementation are iterative processes. The APNs, along with other health care professionals, evaluated the impact of hospital visitation on patient outcomes. The results informed decision makers and were, in part, responsible for a change in local and national policy. In many of the nation's hospitals, therefore, flexible visitation has become the standard of care, and, in many cases, nursing professionals are responsible for quality improvement projects that ensure the standards are implemented.

THE ROLE OF ETHICS IN EVALUATION

Having a solid ethical framework is basic to the APN's role of evaluator. Ethical evaluators systematically and objectively analyze *all* of the information, both positive and negative. Threats to conducting an ethical evaluation may be explicit or implicit (Fitzpatrick et al., 2004). Some common threats are reviewed in this section.

First, an APN may be biased toward an intervention, program, or policy because an APN developed it. If the APN sets out to *prove* that the program works, there is little doubt that the APN will have a hard time being objective. It may be that the APN has put years of labor into implementing a program and believes that it benefits patients. It may be that a great deal of effort has been put into developing these policies, and their implementation has brought professional success. It doesn't matter. Human nature is such that it's very difficult to be unbiased about one's own accomplishments.

Second, an APN may find it hard to be objective because there is administrative support for the program the practitioner has been asked to evaluate. For example, suppose a supervisor has developed a lucrative follow-up program for elderly patients hospitalized with pneumonia. The goal of the program is to decrease future hospitalizations by providing periodic home care. After systematically and objectively examining the program the APN realizes that the frequency of hospitalizations among these patients has not decreased. In a survey, patients say they are generally satisfied receiving care at home, but find the visits to be inconveniently timed and disruptive to the family routine. Some patients report they even enjoy leaving the home on occasion and do not mind keeping clinic appointments. An evaluator might be concerned about reporting these negative results to the administrator.

A third threat relates to structural deficiencies. In the home care example, the practitioner realizes that while administration is touting the benefits of the program, the resources that the hospital provides are inadequate. In order to keep expenses down, the hospital has hired nurses who are not sufficiently qualified and has failed to provide adequate administrative support. Reporting these findings to administration will be a challenge.

There are approaches a practitioner can use when confronted with an explicit or implicit conflict of interest. The APN can discuss the goals and processes of evaluation with an administrator before beginning the study. While working with a team does not always lead to objectivity, a team that includes a member who does not report to the same hospital administrators may also increase the chances of conducting an objective evaluation (Fitzpatrick et al., 2004).

The American Evaluation Association (2004) developed five principles to facilitate ethical conduct for professionals involved in any type of evaluation regardless of the discipline. The first principle focuses on the importance of an objective and systematic examination. The second principle states that the evaluator must be competent. For example, an APN must possess not only advanced nursing skills, but also have the appropriate knowledge and skills needed to conduct an evaluation. Third, evaluators should be honest in planning, implementing, and reporting study results. Fourth, evaluators must respect all individuals and groups including those requesting the evaluation, team members, and patients. Fifth, evaluators must be aware that their responsibility extends to the general public. In conducting the evaluation and reporting the results, they should consider its impact on the cultural and political environment of society.

A MANDATE TO EVALUATE

The mandate to evaluate is integral to professional nursing practice. The focus of the evaluation and the expected competencies will vary based on the educational preparation of the professional nurse. *The Essentials of Master's Education in Nursing* (2011) and *The Essentials of Doctoral Education for Advanced Nursing Practice* (2006), both published by the American Association of Colleges of Nursing (AACN, 2006), outline expectations for advanced nursing practice including evaluation and expected competencies. The documents are organized around specific areas of practice called "Essentials." Each Essential includes a description of the area of practice and related expected competencies. The *Master's Essentials* (Exhibit 1.1) and the *DNP Essentials* (Exhibit 1.2) serve as a blueprint for the education of APNs at their respective levels of advanced practice competencies. Not every Essential includes reference to evaluation; therefore, only those Essentials that address evaluation activities are included in the tables.

EXHIBIT 1.1
The Essentials of Master's Education in Nursing

A number of *The Essentials of Master's Education in Nursing* (2011), henceforth referred to as *MSN Essentials*, address evaluation. The following lists expectations to evaluate by master's prepared nurses as addressed in the specific MSN Essentials.

Essential I: Background for Practice From Sciences and Humanities (AACN, 2011, p. 10)

- Apply ethical analysis and clinical reasoning to assess, intervene, and *evaluate* advanced nursing care delivery
- Use quality processes and improvement sciences to *evaluate* care and ensure patient safety for individuals and communities.

Essential II: Organizational and Systems Leadership (AACN, 2011, p. 12)

- Demonstrate the ability to use complexity science and systems theory in the design, delivery, and *evaluation* of health care.

Essential V: Informatics and Healthcare Technologies (AACN, 2011, p. 19)

- *Evaluate* outcome data, using current communications technologies, information systems, and statistical principles to develop strategies to reduce risks and improvement health outcomes.

Essential VII: Interprofessional Collaboration for Improving Patient and Population Health Outcomes (AACN, 2011, p. 23)

- Employ collaborative strategies in the design, coordination, and *evaluation* of patient-centered care.

Essential VIII: Clinical Prevention and Population Health for Improving Health (AACN, 2011, p. 25)

(continued)

EXHIBIT 1.1 (*continued*)

- *Evaluate* the effectiveness of clinical prevention interventions that affect individual and population-based health outcomes using health information technology and data sources.

Essential IX: Master's-Level Nursing Practice (AACN, 2011, p. 28)

- Apply advanced knowledge of the effects of global environmental, individual, and population characteristics to the design, implementation, and *evaluation* of care.
- Apply knowledge and skills in economics, business principles, and systems in the design, delivery, and *evaluation* of care.
- Apply theory and evidence-based knowledge in leading, as appropriate, the interdisciplinary care team to design, coordinate, and *evaluate* the delivery of patient care.
- Apply learning and teaching principles to the design, implementation, and *evaluation* of health education programs for individuals or groups in a variety of settings.

From American Association of Colleges of Nursing (2011). *The essentials of master's education in nursing.* Washington, DC.

EXHIBIT 1.2
Doctor of Nursing Practice (DNP) Essentials

A number of *The Essentials of Doctoral Education for Advanced Nursing Practice* (2006), henceforth referred to as *DNP Essentials,* also address evaluation. The following lists expectations to evaluate by DNP prepared nurses as addressed in the specific DNP Essential.

Essential I: Scientific Underpinnings for Practice

- Use science-based theories and concept to *evaluate* outcomes.
- Develop and *evaluate* new practice approaches based on nursing theories and theories from other disciplines.

Essential II: Organizational and Systems Leadership for Quality Improvement and Systems Thinking

- *Evaluate* the cost effectiveness of care and use principles of economics and finance to redesign effective and realistic care delivery strategies.
- Develop and *evaluate* care delivery approaches that meet current and future needs of patient populations based on scientific findings in nursing and other clinical sciences, as well as organizational, political, and economic sciences.
- Develop and/or *evaluate* effective strategies for managing the ethical dilemmas inherent in patient care, the health care organization, and research.
- Design, direct, and *evaluate* quality improvement methodologies to promote safe, timely, effective, efficient, equitable, and patient-centered care.

(*continued*)

EXHIBIT 1.2
Doctor of Nursing Practice (DNP) Essentials (*continued*)

Essential III: Clinical Scholarship and Analytical Methods for Evidence-Based Practice

- Design and implement processes to *evaluate* outcomes of practice, practice patterns, and systems of care within a practice setting, health care organization, or community against national benchmarks to determine variances in practice outcomes and population trends.
- Design, direct, and *evaluate* quality improvement methodologies to promote safe, timely, effective, efficient, equitable, and patient-centered care.

Essential IV: Information Systems/Technology and Patient Care Technology for the Improvement and Transformation of Health Care

- Design, select, and use information systems/technology to *evaluate* programs of care, outcomes of care, and care systems.
- Design, select, use, and *evaluate* programs that *evaluate* and monitor outcomes of care, care systems, and quality improvement including consumer use of health care information systems.
- *Evaluate* consumer health information sources for accuracy, timeliness, and appropriateness.

Essential V: Health Care Policy for Advocacy in Health Care

- Develop, *evaluate*, and provide leadership for health care policy that shapes health care financing, regulation, and delivery.

Essential VII: Clinical Prevention and Population Health for Improving the Nation's Health

- *Evaluate* care delivery models and/or strategies using concepts related to community, environmental and occupational health, and cultural and socioeconomic dimensions of health.

Essential VIII: Advanced Nursing Practice

- Design, implement, and *evaluate* therapeutic interventions based on nursing science and other sciences.

From American Association of Colleges of Nursing (2006). *The essentials of doctoral education for advanced nursing practice.* Washington, DC.

QUALITY AND SAFETY EDUCATION FOR NURSES PROJECT

The overall goal of the Quality and Safety Education for Nurses (QSEN) project, funded by the Robert Wood Johnson Foundation (RWJF) is to meet the challenge of preparing future nurses with the knowledge, skills, and attitudes (KSAs) necessary to continuously improve the quality and safety of the health care systems in which they work. The project has examined nursing education from a contemporary quality and safety perspective and has published competencies for baccalaureate-prepared nurses and APNs without differentiating the APN based on master's or doctoral preparation (Cronenwett et al., 2009). A landmark report, *Health Professions Education: A Bridge to Quality* (Institute of Medicine [IOM], 2003), identified competencies that all health professional must have for practice in the 21st century. These five competencies address the basis for all health professionals to provide patient-centered care, work in interdisciplinary teams, employ evidence-based practice, utilize quality improvement methodologies, and integrate informatics in providing care. The QSEN project has built on these five competencies and has added safety as the sixth competency to their framework. Expected competencies related to evaluation are addressed in the QSEN framework and are listed in Exhibit 1.3.

It is clear from these important publications and others as well, that there is a clear mandate for evaluation by APNs regardless of the setting, population, or focus of service.

SUMMARY

This chapter acquainted the APN with the basic concepts and definitions related to evaluation, and highlighted the expectation to evaluate within the Essentials documents for master's education and doctor of nursing practice education. The message is clear that APNs are responsible and accountable to conduction evaluations. The fundamental purpose of evaluation is to provide information for decision making. Within the backdrop of a developing body of knowledge about evaluation, the APN must understand what is possible methodologically and what outcomes one can expect.

There are many ways to conduct evaluations, and professional evaluators tend to agree that there is no "one best way" to do any evaluation. Instead, good evaluation requires carefully thinking through the questions that need to be answered, the type of program being evaluated, and the way

EXHIBIT 1.3
Quality and Safety Education for Nurses (QSEN) Project

Evidence-Based Practice:
- *Evaluate* organization cultures and structures that promote evidence-based practice.

Safety:
- *Evaluate* effective strategies to reduce reliance on memory.

Informatics:
- *Evaluate* the strengths and weaknesses of information systems used in patient care.
- *Evaluate* benefits and limitations of different communication technologies and their impact on safety and quality.

in which the information generated will be used. "Good evaluation should provide useful information about program functioning that can contribute to program improvement" (Kellogg, 2004). For good program planning, monitoring, and evaluation, it is important to know not only what the program expects to achieve, but also how it achieves those outcomes. The evaluator must understand the principles on which a program is based (Weiss, 1998). Discussions about the *whethers, hows,* and *whys* of program success require credible evidence and attention to the paths by which outcomes and impacts are produced. Subsequent chapters will lead the APN down a path to increase understanding of evaluations in specific areas of interest in health care.

REFERENCES

American Association of Colleges of Nursing. (2006). *The essentials of doctoral education for advanced nursing practice.* Washington, DC: Author.

American Association of Colleges of Nursing. (2011). *The essentials of master's education in nursing.* Washington, DC: Author.

American Evaluation Association. (2004). *Guiding principles for evaluators.* Fairhaven, MA: American Evaluation Association. Retrieved from http://www.eval.org/Publications/GuidingPrinciples.asp

American Nurses Association. (2010). *Nursing: Scope and standards of practice* (2nd ed.). Washington, DC: Author.

Anderson, L. W., & Krathwohl, D. R. (Eds.). (2001). *A taxonomy for learning, teaching, and assessing: A revision of Bloom's taxonomy of educational objectives.* New York, NY: Longman.

Archives of the American College of Surgeons. *History and archives of the American College of Surgeons: Ernest A. Codman.* Retrieved from http://www.facs.org/archives/monthly highlight.html

Barrett-Connor, E., Grady, D., & Stefanick, M. L. (2005). The rise and fall of menopausal hormone therapy. *Annual Review of Public Health, 26,* 115–140. doi:101146/annurev.publhealth.26.021304.144637

Benner, P., Hughes, R. G., & Sutphen, M. (2008). Clinical reasoning, decision-making, and action: Thinking critically and clinically. In R. G. Hughes (Ed.), *Patient safety and quality: An evidence-based handbook for nurses* (Vol. 1, pp. 87–109). Rockville, MD: Agency for Healthcare Research and Quality.

Bloom, B., Enlerhart, M., Furst, E., Hill, W., & Krathwohl, D. (1956). *Taxonomy of educational objectives: The classification of educational goals. Handbook I: Cognitive domain.* New York, NY: Longmans, Green.

Bloom, M., Fischer, J., & Orme, J. G. (1999). *Evaluating practice-guidelines for the accountable professional.* Needham Heights, MA: Allyn & Bacon.

Brook, R. H., & Lohr, K. N. (1985). Efficacy, effectiveness, variations, and quality. Boundary crossing research. *Medical Care, 23*(5), 710–722.

Casarett, D., Karlawish, J. H. T., & Sugarman, J. (2000). Determining when quality improvement initiatives should be considered research: Proposed criteria and potential implications. *JAMA, 282*(17), 2275–2280.

Centers for Disease Control and Prevention. (1999). *Defining public health research and public health non-research.* Retrieved from http://www.cdc.gov/od/science/regs/hrpp/research definition.htm

Codman, E. A. (2009). The registry of bone sarcomas as an example of the end-result idea in hospital organization. *Clinical Orthopaedics and Related Research, 467,* 2766–2770. doi: 10.1007/s11999-009-1048-7

Cronenwett, L., Sherwood, G., Pohl, J., Barnsteiner, J., Moore, S., & Sullivan, D., & Warren, J. (2009). Quality and safety education for advanced nursing practice. *Nursing Outlook, 57*(6), 338–348.

DeLeskey, K. (2009). Family visitation in the PACU: The current state of practice in the United States. *Journal of PeriAnesthesia Nursing, 24*(2), 81–85.

Donabedian, A. (1980). *Explorations in quality assessment and monitoring. Vol. 1. The definition of quality and approaches to its assessment.* Ann Arbor, MI: Health Administration Press.

Donabedian, A. (1982). *Explorations in quality assessment and monitoring. Vol. 2. The criteria and standards of quality.* Ann Arbor, MI: Health Administration Press.

Donabedian, A. (1989). The end results of health care: Ernest Codman's contribution to quality assessment and beyond. *The Milbank Quarterly, 67*(2), 233–261.

Donabedian, A. (2003a). *An introduction to quality assurance in health care.* New York, NY: Oxford University Press.

Donabedian, A. (2003b). *An introduction to quality assurance in health care* (p. xxiii). New York, NY: Oxford University Press.

Drummond, M. F., Sculpher, M. J., Torrance. G. W., O'Briend, B. J., & Stoddart, G. L. (2005). *Methods for the economic evaluation of health care programmes.* Oxford, UK: Oxford University Press.

Fitzpatrick, J. L., Sanders, J. R., & Worthen, B. R. (2004). *Program evaluation. Alternative approaches and practical guidelines.* Boston, MA: Pearson Education, Inc.

Frazier, A., Frazier, H., & Warren, N. A. (2010). A discussion of family-centered care within the pediatric intensive care unit. *Critical Care Nursing Quarterly, 33*(1), 82–86.

Guralnik, D. B. (1979). *Webster's new world dictionary of the American language.* New York, NY: Simon and Schuster.

Hersch, A. L., Stefanick, M. L., & Stafford, R. S. (2004). National use of postmeno-pausal hormone therapy. *JAMA, 291*(1), 47–53.

Hulley, S., Grady, D., Bush, E., Furberg, C. Herrington, D., Riggs, B., & Vittinghoff, E. (1998). Randomized trial of estrogen plus progestin for secondary prevention of coronary heart disease in postmenopausal women. Heart and Estrogen/Progestin Replacement Study (HERS) Research Group. *JAMA, 280*(7), 605–613.

Institute of Medicine. (1990). *Medicare: A strategy for quality assurance* (Vol. 1). Washington, DC: National Academy Press.

Institute of Medicine. (2003). *Health professions education: A bridge to quality.* Washington, DC: National Academies Press.

Kamerling, S. N., Lawler, L. C., Lynch, M., & Schwartz, A. J. (2008). Family-centered care in the pediatric post anesthesia care unit: Changing practice to promote parental visitation. *Journal of PeriAnesthesia Nursing, 23*(1), 5–16.

Kellogg, W. K. (2004). *Logic model development guide.* Battle Creek, MI: W. K. Kellogg Foundation.

Maurer, F., & Smith, C. M. (2004). *Community/public health nursing.* St Louis, MO: Elsevier.

McNett, M., & Lawry, K. (2009). Research and quality improvement activities: When is institutional review board review needed? *Journal of Neuroscience Nursing, 41*(6), 344–347.

Merriam-Webster Dictionary. Retrieved from www.merriam-webster.com/dictionary

Miller, F. G., & Emanuel, E. J. (2008). Quality-improvement research and informed consent. *New England Journal of Medicine, 358*(8), 765–767.

Morris, P. A., & Dracup, K. (2007). Quality improvement or research? The ethics of hospital project oversight. *American Journal of Critical Care, 16*, 424–426.

Mulley, A. G. (1989). E. A. Codman and the end results idea: A commentary. *The Milbank Quarterly, 67*(2), 257–261.

Nelson, E. C., Batalden, P. B., & Godfrey, M. M. (2007). *Quality by design: A clinical microsystems approach.* San Francisco, CA: Jossey-Bass.

Newhouse, R. P. (2007). Diffusing confusion among evidence-based practice, quality improvement, and research. *JONA, 37*(10), 432–435.

Nightingale, F. (1859). *Notes on nursing.* USA: ReadaClassic.com. (Reproduced in 2010.)

Obama, B. (2010, April 15). *Presidential memorandum-hospital visitation.* Washington, DC: The White House. Retrieved from http://www.whitehouse.gov/the-press-office/presidential-memorandum-hospital-visitation

Powazek, M., Goff, J. R., Schyving, J., & Paulson, M. A. (1978). Emotional reactions of children to isolation in a cancer hospital. *Journal of Pediatrics, 92*(5), 834–837.

Reinhardt, A. C., & Ray, L. N. (2003). Differentiating quality improvement from research. *Applied Nursing Research, 16*(1), 2–8.

Robert Wood Johnson Foundation. Glossary of health care quality terms. Retrieved from http://www.rwjf.org/qualityequity/glossary.jsp?

Rossouw, J. E., Anderson, G. L., Prentice, R. L., LaCroix, A. Z., Kooperberg, C., Stefanick, M. L., ... Ockene, J. (2002). Risks and benefits of estrogen plus progestin in healthy postmenopausal women: Principal results from the women's health Initiative randomized controlled trial. *JAMA, 288*(3), 321–333.

Sidani, S., & Braden, C. J. (1998). *Evaluating nursing interventions: A theory-driven approach.* Thousand Oaks, CA: Sage Publications.

Spiegelhalter, D. J. (1999). Surgical audit: Statistical lessons from Nightingale and Codman. *Journal of the Royal Statistical Society, A, 162*(Pt. 1), 45–58.

Sunōl, R. (2000). Avedis Donabedian. *International Journal for Quality in Health Care, 12*(6), 451–454.

U.S. Department of Health & Human Services. (2009, January 5). *Office for Human Research Protections (OHRP). OHRP Quality Improvement Frequently Asked Questions.* Retrieved from http://www.hhs.gov/ohrp/qualityfaq.html

Walls, M. (2009). Staff attitudes and beliefs regarding family visitation after implementation of a formal visitation policy in the PACU. *Journal of PeriAnesthesia Nursing, 24*(4), 229–232.

Weiss, C. H. (1998). *Evaluations: Methods for studying programs and policies* (2nd ed.). Upper Saddle River, NJ: Prentice Hall.

TWO

The Nature of Evidence as a Basis for Evaluation

Joanne V. Hickey

"It ain't so much what you don't know that gets you into trouble, it's what you know for sure that just ain't so."

Mark Twain

INTRODUCTION

Evaluation is based on collecting, analyzing, organizing, and critically reviewing evidence to make a judgment or decision about value. This chapter will define evidence from a generic perspective and will discuss the sources of evidence in its many forms. It will describe how evidence is organized and ranked, will address evidence integrity, and will examine how evidence is used and interpreted for evaluation. This information will provide a basis for exploring how APNs acquire and use evidence for evaluation. The chapter is organized around a broad discussion of evidence and then focuses on the use of evidence by APNs. Evidence, within the context of evidence-based practice in patient centered clinical practice, will be discussed in Chapter 7.

BASIC CONCEPTS FROM LOGIC AND EPISTEMOLOGY

A number of terms are threaded into the discussion about evidence such as proposition, inference, premise, induction, deduction, and conclusion. A *proposition* is a statement or declarative sentence that may be true or false. *Inference* is a logical or conceptual process of deriving a statement from one or more other statements (Angeles, 1992, p. 145). For example, because large organizations are complex and the organization under review is large, it is reasonable to assume that the organization under review is complex. A *premise* is defined as a statement that is true or that is believed to be true; it is any statement that serves as the basis for an argument or inference (Angeles, 1992, p. 240). A premise is composed of propositions; when taken together, they form a conclusion. For example, intensive care units within the same facility sometimes have different lengths of stay. Yet these units are part of the same organization. One can surmise that patient acuity and practice patterns must play some part in determining length of stay.

Induction is the process of reasoning from a part to a whole, from a particular instant of something to a general statement, or from particular to universal (Angeles, 1992, p. 144). For example, if using a particular patient-turning device on one unit of a facility is effective in reducing pressure ulcers, then using the device on all other units in the facility should also be effective in reducing pressure ulcers throughout the facility. This statement may or may not be true for a variety of reasons such as variations in patient populations and acuity. *Deduction* is the process of reasoning from a general truth to a particular instant of a truth, from the general to the particular, or from the universal to the particular. For example, all men have two feet and two arms; John is a man; therefore, John has two feet and two arms. A *conclusion* is a statement that has been inferred from other statements. It is the logical consequence or implication of the premises of an argument (Angeles, 1992, p. 51).

Evidence

To have evidence is to have some conceptual warrant for belief or action (Goodman, 2003, p. 2). Basing all beliefs and practices strictly on evidence allegedly separates science from other activities (Husserl, 1982; Kuhn, 1996). For APNs, the word evidence is usually synonymous with evidence-based practice. However, evidence is a broader and generic concept that can be a noun or a verb. For purposes of this discussion, only evidence as a noun is addressed. According to Webster's, evidence is a condition of being evident; something that makes another thing evident; and something that tends to prove or to provide grounds for belief. It is that which is accepted as conclusive (e.g., clear, obvious, acceptable, confirmed) support of a statement (Angeles, 1992, p. 97). Evidence has also been defined as:

- The basis of belief; the substantiation or confirmation that is needed in order to believe that something is true (Pearson, Wiechula, Court, & Lockwood, 2005).
- The available facts and circumstances supporting, or otherwise, a belief or proposition, or indicating whether a thing is true or valid (Pearsall & Trumble, 1995).

From a legal perspective, evidence is something presented in a legal proceeding; it is a statement of a witness. Further investigation of a variety of websites uncovers the following definitions: Evidence is that which tends to prove or disprove something; grounds for belief; proof; something that makes plain or clear; and an indication or sign. From law, evidence is data presented to a court or jury in proof of the facts about something; it may include the testimony of witnesses, records, documents, or objects (http://dictionary. reference.com/browse/evidence-9-24-10). Synonyms often used for evidence are information, knowledge, exhibit, testimony, and proof.

Review of subcategories of evidence from law offers insight into concepts useful for this discussion. For example, *clear and convincing evidence* is evidence demonstrating a high probability of truth of the factual matter under review. This definition suggests the need for high-level, reliable, and valid information, as well as some system of ranking of evidence. *Corroborating evidence* is evidence that is independent of and different from other evidence, but supplements and strengthens evidence already presented as proof. In evaluation, different kinds of information are collected from a variety of sources to provide a comprehensive view to assist the evaluator in making judgments. Sources of evidence from a variety of sources provide for triangulation of information. *Cumulative evidence* is additional evidence that is similar to evidence already presented as proof of the same factual matter. Collecting information over time elucidates trends and consistencies or inconsistencies important in evaluation. *Demonstrative evidence* is evidence in the form of objects (e.g., diagrams, models, tables) that is used to illustrate and clarify the factual matter presented. The evaluator is often responsible for synthesizing large amounts of information and presenting it in a concise and understandable form for other decision makers. Crunching of information through diagrams, dashboards, models, and other presentation strategies are commonly used. *Relevant evidence* is evidence that tends to prove or disprove an issue of fact that is of consequence to the work or project.

The evaluator is challenged to search and find the best information important to the project. This requires comprehensive knowledge about collecting targeted information through a variety of sources such as electronic databases, expert consultation, and other repositories of information. In the pursuit of the "best evidence" to evaluate anything—a program, practice change, or published guidelines—evaluation is a high-level, complex process that involves an understanding of the nature of evidence and how it is used and evaluated as a basis for decision making. In evaluation, evidence can be considered clues or pieces of a puzzle that contribute to creating an accurate picture of the focus of evaluation. It is a process to search for truth as a basis for evaluation.

Data, Information, Knowledge, and Understanding

The words data, information, knowledge, and understanding are often used interchangeably in practice and evaluation. According to Graves and Corcoran (1989) *datum* (singular; data, plural) is a single entity that has been described objectively and has not been interpreted. An example of datum is a single blood pressure or apical pulse value. *Information* is defined as data that have been interpreted, organized, or structured (American Nurses Association [ANA], 2001). An example of information is an evaluator noticing a trend in gradually rising systolic blood pressure when a 48-hour period of time is reviewed. *Knowledge* is defined as information that has been synthesized so that relationships are identified and formalized (ANA, 2001). An example of knowledge is realizing that the rising systolic blood pressure in a brain-injured patient could be a sign of increased intracranial pressure.

A review of the framework proposed by Ackoff (1989) helps differentiate data, information, and knowledge. He proposed that the content of the human mind can be classified into five categories: data, information, knowledge, understanding, and wisdom. In addition to defining data, information, and knowledge, he also included the terms understanding and wisdom. These terms are described in Table 2.1. *Understanding* is described as a cognitive and analytical process of applying and appreciating relationships. *Wisdom* has many definitions that include an ethical and moral tone. Frances Hutcheson said that wisdom denotes the pursuit of the best ends by the best means (Knowles, 1999, p. 396).

In describing the Achoff model, Bellinger, Castro, and Mills (2004) note that the first four categories are related to the past and address what has happened or what is known. The fifth category, wisdom, focuses on the future because it incorporates vision and design. With wisdom, the future can be created, thus extending vision and understanding of the past and present.

Rycroft-Malone et al. (2004) provide an interesting discussion about knowledge. Knowledge has been divided into *propositional* and *non-propositional knowledge* (Eraut, 1985; 2000; see Table 2.2 for a comparison). By formal-explicit versus informal-implicit is meant that formal-explicit characteristics of propositional knowledge come from organized knowledge derived from rigorous research methods that can be generalized and disseminated through publications, presentations, and other media. By comparison, the informal-implicit characteristics of non-propositional knowledge come from professional- and discipline-specific and personal knowledge that an individual brings to a particular situation without the primary purpose of transferability (Eraut, 2000; Higgs & Titchen, 1995). Non-propositional knowledge may become propositional knowledge as the tacit knowledge accumulates and is tested using rigorous research methodologies yielding results that can then become generalizable. Although knowledge based on research with the resulting propositional knowledge has been viewed as higher-level knowledge than non-propositional knowledge, it is becoming clearer that both categories of knowledge are needed working together in synergy to provide the most comprehensive collection of evidence for understanding.

TABLE 2.1

Data, Information, Knowledge, Understanding, and Wisdom Model

Term	Definition/Description	Example
Data	Symbols Exists in and of itself and has no significance beyond its existence Does not have meaning by itself Exists in both usable and non-usable forms	Single blood pressure, pulse, or serum glucose reading Overall budget amount
Information	Data that are processed and have been given meaning by way of connecting them to something The meaning provided may or may not be useful Provides answers to "who," "what," "where," and "when" questions	Notice of trend in decrease in satisfaction score after elimination of receptionist in clinic
Knowledge	Application of data and information Collection of information organized to be useful It is not at the level of integration Provides answers to how something works Answers "how" questions	Recognizing the fit of using complexity science as a framework to understanding implementation of electronic medical records in a health care organization
Understanding	A cognitive and analytical process of applying and appreciating relationships Process by which knowledge can be synthesized into new knowledge by combining other knowledge with current knowledge to create something new	A teacher understands the relationship between using multiple methods of instruction and particular learning styles of students in mastering competencies

(continued)

TABLE 2.1
Data, Information, Knowledge, Understanding, and Wisdom Mode (*continued*)

Term	Definition/Description	Example
Wisdom	Evaluated understanding based on an integration and synthesis of cumulative knowledge and experience and inclusion of a moral and ethical context to provide insight and high level understanding to complex and not easily answered questions	Ability to appreciate the ethical and moral impact of providing access to care for all members of a society

Empiricism and Positivism

Historically, evidence has its roots in empiricism and positivism, a philosophical view that has greatly influenced the perceptions of knowledge in nursing for decades (Billay, Myrick, Luhanga, & Yonge, 2007). *Empiricism* is a branch of philosophy that ties knowledge to experience. It states that all ideas are abstractions formed by combining and recombining what is experienced. Experience is the sole source of knowledge, and all that we know is ultimately dependent upon sense data. Information provided by our senses serves as the basic building block for all knowledge (Angeles, 1992, p. 85). Positivism is an outgrowth of traditional empiricism attributed to Comte, the 19th century French philosopher, and is based on the belief that the highest or only form of knowledge is the description of sensory phenomena. Comte expounded three stages of human belief: the theological; the metaphysical; and the positive. Positivism was so named because it confined itself to what is positively given,

TABLE 2.2
Comparison of Propositional Knowledge and Non-Propositional Knowledge

Propositional Knowledge	Non-Propositional Knowledge
Formal	Informal
Explicit	Implicit
Derived from research and scholarly work	Derived primarily from practice
Focused on generalizability	Focused on an individual; linked to experience and cognition resources of an individual

thus avoiding all speculation (Blackburn, 2008, p. 283). From a positivist perspective, knowledge is equated to truth that can be discovered.

From an empirical framework, evidence comes exclusively from one's experiences. What one sees, hears, and feels through touch, smells, or tastes are interpreted and that interpretation is one's source of knowledge and the evidence for making sense of everything. Yet, an empirical approach to evidence and knowledge is dependent upon a number of interrelated factors that include: what we experience as we live; awareness of that experience; how we process and think about the experience (perception); how we talk about that experience; and how we diagram or sketch the experience. Therefore, the sources of evidence based on empiricism are personal observation and experience along with one's interpretation of those observations or experiences. An example of current work grounded in empirical tradition is exemplified by the definition of evidence provided by Guyatt, Rennie, Meade, and Cook who have published extensively about evidence-based practice. They define evidence as an empirical observation that constitutes potential evidence whether systematically collected or not (Guyatt, Rennie, Meade, & Cook, 2008). Copi and Cohen (2009), in their book on logic, note that evidence ultimately refers to experience.

Many would argue that this is a narrow perspective of evidence for the 21st century and is prone to bias, which will be discussed later in this chapter. Goldberg (2006) argues that rather than empirical evidence increasing certainty by factoring out the subjective and contextual components of every-day experience that bias understanding, empirical evidence obscures the subjective elements that inescapably enter all forms of human inquiry. From this perspective evidence is not objective or neutral, but rather part of a social system of knowledge production. Although health professionals have been taught to value empirical knowledge above all forms of knowledge, new paradigms are challenging these beliefs and are redefining how health professionals think about the bases of health care and practice.

Another approach to evidence is to examine how we know. Carper (1978), in a seminal article, described four fundamental patterns of knowing in nursing. The first pattern of knowing is *empirical knowledge*. The basis of this pattern is positivism, "which believes that objective data, measurement, and generalizability are essential to the generation and dissemination of [nursing] knowledge" (Streubert-Speziale & Carpenter, 2003, p. 4). An example of empirical knowing is knowledge from the physical and biological sciences that help nurses to understand laws of movement and human physiology. The second pattern of knowing is *aesthetics*. It involves the subjective experience and the creative aspect of nursing care. This concept is more difficult to define, but Fawcett et al. (2001, p. 6) propose that aesthetic knowing is "the 'artful' performance of manual and technical skills." It answers the question of "how" a nursing act is performed rather than the key elements of the act. Aesthetic knowing has to do with style and delivery, which is personalized by the nurse for a particular patient. The third way of knowing is *personal knowing*, which involves the nurse as a person. The nurse is present or connects with others, a process often referred to as the therapeutic nurse-patient relationship (Fawcett et al., 2001) or intersubjectivity, the subject-to-subject relationship involving true presence (Parse, 1981, 1992). Presence refers to being totally focused and "being there" with authenticity and honesty in open, honest, and genuine communications. The fourth way of knowing is *ethical knowing* and addresses the ethical and moral component of practice. It guides the nurse about how to behave in a given situation and emanates from an individual's sense of right and wrong. It requires the nurse to understand various philosophical perspectives and accepted standards of conduct and practice regarding what is good, right, and desirable (Billay et al., 2007).

Other scholars have added to Carper's work including White (1995) who suggested that the fifth way of knowing is *sociopolitical* knowing. This form of knowing relates to how nurses address cultural differences of patients, political awareness, and policy issues and adds to the contextual component of individualized care. What is clear from this brief overview of knowing is that no single pattern of knowing should be used in isolation from the others because the practice of nursing relies on all five ways of knowing to provide quality care. Knowing is a form of the stream of evidence that guides practice including the dimension of evaluation.

Other Perspectives About Knowledge

Empiricism and positivism have had critics beginning with philosophers such as Dewey and others who believed that knowledge was not something that must correspond to some antecedent truth, super-imposed reality, or predefined description of the world, but rather knowledge is something emergent that is always interactive with experience and action, and as such, requires continuous interpretation or revised description (Mantzoukas, 2007). Mantzoukas goes on to say that knowledge is inextricably linked with action, and is specific, with good action described as that which works and is effective. Knowledge and advancement of knowledge emerge from our interpretive descriptions of the effectiveness or not of our experiences and actions (Gallagher, 1964). Building on the concept that knowledge emerges from actions and practice experiences, Schon (1983) proposed the concept of reflection as a means for acquiring and developing professional knowledge. Schon (1983, 1987) reasoned that research-based knowledge driven by theory resulted in linear, certain, and clear-cut solutions. By comparison, practice is non-linear, uncertain, complex, and conflicting. Therefore, positivism-based research knowledge does not provide all of the answers to practitioners and does not guarantee best practice.

Practitioners need to use reflective techniques to identify and frame unique problematic situations and find workable unique solutions. By consciously analyzing the problematic situation and action taken, lessons can inform future practice about what works and what is more effective. Refection offers a means for explicating practice, analyzing decision-making processes, and ensuring individualized and unique best practice and care. Reflection is described as a process of transforming unconscious types of knowledge and practices into conscious, explicit, and logically articulated knowledge and practices that allow for transparent and justifiable clinical decision making (Freshwater, Taylor, & Sherwood, 2008; Johns & Freshwater, 2005; Mantzoukas, 2007).

Nursing's thought leaders have built on the concept of reflection in many ways including intuitive knowledge in nursing practice. Mitchell (1994) defines intuition as the instant understanding of knowledge without evidence of sensible thought. In addressing clinical intuition, Benner and Tanner (1987) write that intuition is understanding without rationale. Intuition is a process of arriving at accurate conclusions based on relatively small amounts of knowledge and/or information (Westcott, cited in Benner & Tanner, 1968). In the renowned book, *From Novice to Expert: Excellence and Power in Clinical Nursing Practice* (1984), Benner reports on research that investigated how nurses make clinical decisions based on different levels of experience. The levels of nursing practice are novice, advanced beginner, competent, proficient, and expert. Inherent in the notion of the expert nurse is intuitive knowing, which is also called intuitive knowledge. It is intuitive knowledge and judgment that separates expert judgment from that of a beginner (Benner & Tanner, 1987, p. 23). According to Benner and other nurse scholars, intuition is a source of knowledge in nursing to be valued and embraced. Some authors refer to intuition as tacit knowledge. *Tacit knowledge* is defined as "a state of a person or a relation between people that is not expressed, or one of which the subject may be unaware, but which can be inferred from their other capacities or activities" (Blackburn, 2008, p. 358). Blackburn (2008, p. 358) also defines *tacit communications* as the unexpressed recognition of the position of others that leads to strategies from common activity. It is knowledge that is so embedded and integrated into one's thinking that there may not even be conscious awareness of its presence.

Reflection provides structure and guidance to transpose unconscious and intuitive types of knowledge to conscious knowledge and allows for linkages to be developed with previous knowledge and experience, formal theories, and research knowledge to provide the best sources of evidence for professional practice and care.

SOURCES OF EVIDENCE

To answer the question, where does evidence come from, there are many ways to think about the sources of evidence. One way to classify the sources of evidence is by primary, secondary, and tertiary sources. *Primary sources* of evidence refer to information in its original form. That is, information that has not been interpreted, condensed, or evaluated. It is the original thinking, reports, discoveries, or shared new insights. Primary sources represent the first time the material has been released in physical, print or electronic, format. Examples of primary sources include journal articles published in peer review journals; survey results; proceedings of meetings, conferences, or symposia; newspaper or electronic media postings; patient medical records; and data sets such as national census descriptive statistics (University of Maryland Libraries, 2006). *Secondary sources* of evidence are accounts that are removed from the event or information and are provided after the fact. They describe, interpret, analyze, or evaluate information provided from primary sources. Examples of secondary sources are biographies, commentaries, monographs, textbooks, review articles, critiques, or opinion articles. *Tertiary sources* of evidence are works that include both primary and secondary resources in a special subject area that have been synthesized, reformatted, and condensed to a convenient and easy-to-read format. It may also include compilations of primary and secondary sources of information that recommend how to use the information. Examples of tertiary sources are clinical guidelines, manuals, handbooks, and practice protocols.

The sources of evidence can come from external and internal sources. *External evidence* is generated through rigorous research such as randomized controlled trials and can be generalized to other settings. Melnyk and Fineout-Overholt (2011) point out that an important question to consider when applying external evidence to a project is that the same results are achieved that were reported in the research. In other words, does the research evidence translate and transfer to a real-world setting and project? By contrast, *internal evidence* is evidence generated through practice initiatives such as outcomes management and quality improvement projects that were conducted to improve care or outcomes in the setting in which the change was initiated.

Another way to think about the sources of evidence is based on qualitative and quantitative methods. *Qualitative methods* are used to investigate a phenomenon or area of interest through the collection of (non-numeric) narrative materials using a variety of methods to collect the data. By comparison, *quantitative methods* collect data in a quantified (numeric) form; the focus of the investigation lends itself to precise measurement and quantification. This raises the question of value. Is evidence from one method of investigation better when conducting an evaluation? The response to that question is, it depends. It depends upon the elements of the evaluation and what evidence you are trying to collect. Some questions are answerable by qualitative methods. For example, if the evaluator wishes to determine how staff nurses feel about having a seminal event in a clinical unit, then qualitative methods such as semi-structured interviews would be appropriate to tap into those personal responses. However, if the evaluator wishes to determine the demographic characteristics of the nursing staff employed in a cardiovascular service, then quantitative methods such as a forced-choice questionnaire would be appropriate. In most evaluations, both qualitative and quantitative methods are needed to collect all of the evidence necessary to complete a comprehensive evaluation.

Still another perspective about the sources of evidence is practitioner-generated evidence called reflective knowledge, previously discussed in this chapter. The fundamental basis of reflection is primarily the experiences of the practitioner and the conscious effort of the practitioner to link this reflective knowledge with other types of knowledge to be applied to the current situation of interest. Understanding reflective knowledge and how it is used in practice and evaluation is complex and slowly evolving.

QUALITY OF EVIDENCE

Quality is a notion that has to do with value to the beholder, thus suggesting a degree of subjectivity. The quality of evidence can be examined from a number of perspectives. Because evaluation is based on the accumulation and organization of evidence, examining the quality of evidence is briefly addressed in this section.

Bias, Validity, and Reliability of Evidence

In examining the quality of evidence in any evaluation, bias, validity, and reliability, which influence evidence and its usefulness in the evaluation process, must be considered. For the purposes of this chapter, *bias* is defined as any influence that produces a distortion in the result of an evaluation. It can affect the quality of evidence in both qualitative and quantitative components of an evaluation (Polit & Beck, 2008, p. 197). Bias can be further divided into bias related to the evaluator or observer and bias related to evidence and process.

Evaluator/Observer Bias

Evaluator bias can occur in a number of forms. If the evaluator interviews people in the course of the evaluation process, interviewer bias is possible. The ideal interviewer is a neutral agent through which evaluation-focused questions are passed and recorded. However, this seemingly simple notion is difficult to achieve. The respondents and interviewer interact on a human level that includes complex verbal and non-verbal communications and interactions. These interactions can affect the interviewee's responses to questions. This means the quality of the information or evidence provided is inaccurate or incomplete, thus having a negative effect on the evaluation outcome. Evaluator bias may be communicated verbally or non-verbally, and the bias may be subtle. The basis of the bias may be personal preference for the outcome of the evaluation, allegiances to stakeholders who will be affected by the evaluation outcome, or a desire to validate previously articulated beliefs or experience.

A second potential source of evaluator bias is *observer bias*; that is, the evaluator collects evidence for an evaluation by observation. Observation is often an excellent alternative to self-reporting methods with subjects. Observation is useful to record characteristics and conditions of individuals, groups, and environments; verbal and non-verbal communications; activities and behaviors; and performance characteristics. Polit and Beck (2008, p. 370) address factors that interfere with objective observations; they include the following:

- Observer prejudices, attitudes, and values may result in faulty inferences.
- Personal interest and commitment may distort observations in a preferred direction.
- Anticipation of what is to be observed may affect what is observed.
- Premature decisions before adequate evidence is collected may result in errors of classification or conclusions.

Although observational biases cannot be removed completely, they can be minimized through the careful training of the observer and attention to bias in the study design. Structured observations help to control bias and to systematically record observations so that comparable evidence is collected for all subjects.

Participant Bias

As with evaluator bias, there is potential bias from the participants in an evaluation. In any evaluation, evidence is often collected from people either directly or indirectly involved in the evaluation process. Participants may be a source of evidence through input from interviews or from information provided though questionnaires, documents, reports, or other sources of evidence. Bias can be introduced in a number of ways such as *non-response bias*, *selection bias*, and *attrition bias*. Individuals decide if they wish to participate in an evaluation. It is important for the evaluator to determine if there are any group differences between the responders and non-responders, such as demographic, socioeconomic, or other differences, that could be a source of bias. This form of bias is called *non-response bias*. Another form of bias is *selection bias*. The evaluator must have a representative sample to collect evidence so that there is no segment of evidence excluded from the evaluation that could distort the findings. *Attrition bias* refers to participants who remove themselves from continuation in the process. The evaluator should determine if there are any group differences between those that continue to participate and those who withdraw. The reasons for withdrawal may provide important insight about the evaluation or the evaluation process. Participants who are directly interviewed by the evaluator may demonstrate social desirability response bias, and extreme response bias. *Social desirability response bias* is noted when participants mask their responses consistently and provide responses that are reflective of prevailing social values or professional expectations (Polit & Beck, 2008, p. 432). Another form of social desirability bias occurs when the respondent knows or has a personal relationship with the evaluator. The respondent may not wish to offend the evaluator or may not wish the responses to seem critical or unappreciative of the evaluator's efforts, so the respondent may answer in a way that he or she believes will please, or at least not offend, the evaluator. *Extreme response bias* is demonstrated by participants who distort their opinions and respond so that everything is reported as very positive or very negative. In designing an evaluation, the evaluator should take into consideration all possible sources of bias and attempt to find ways to control or minimize their influence.

Validity

Validity is often associated with the research literature. Evaluation is a form of research, especially when it is conducted with the rigor of a scientific investigation. Many concepts addressed in research texts are applicable to evaluation. From the perspective of research design, Shadish, Cook, and Campbell (2002, p. 34) define validity as, "the approximate truth of an inference." Polit and Beck (2008) note that validity is not an absolute value, but a matter of degree. Moving from a perspective of validity in research to evidence, *validity of evidence* is the degree to which the evidence is justified, supported, and founded on truth. Therefore, the validity of evidence is critical when considering design, conduct, and analysis in evaluation.

In research parlance, validity is subdivided into internal validity and external validity. *Internal validity* is defined as the extent to which one can make an inference that the independent variable is influencing the dependent variable and that the relationship is not spurious (Polit & Beck, 2008, p. 295). *External validity* is defined as a state in which the results can confidently be generalized to situations outside the specific evaluation setting (Polit & Beck, 2008, p. 295). There are a number of threats to internal validity that include temporal ambiguity, selection, history, maturation, mortality/attrition, and testing/instrumentation. These concepts are well described in a number of research texts and will not be addressed in this chapter.

A special form of validity, called construct validity, is an important consideration in evaluation. A *construct* is an abstract (non-observable) entity, the existence of which is postulated and explained by use of observable phenomena (Angeles, 1992, p. 55). *Construct validity* is the inferences from the particulars of a study to the higher-order constructs that they are intended to represent (Polit & Beck, 2008, p. 299). The concept of construct validity can also be applied to evaluation. Constructs link the methods used in the evaluation to the higher order concept of interest and to the ways the resulting evidence is translated into knowledge to make decisions related to that concept. A construct in an evaluation must be defined and operationalized before the evaluator can decide what the key characteristics of interest are and what is the best way to measure those characteristics. For example, if the focus of the evaluation is to examine interdisciplinary collaboration on a unit, the evaluator must first describe and operationalize the concept of interdisciplinary collaboration. What are the key characteristics to examine? A review of the literature might reveal that interdisciplinary collaboration is based on mutual respect, transparency, open and honest communications, and a common goal. The evaluator would then focus on ways to collect evidence about these attributes from the team that is being evaluated. As there are a variety of methods of eliciting the evidence related to a construct, the evaluator would have to decide what methods would provide the best evidence to address the question. The evaluator may use more than one method to collect evidence, which is often necessary to provide information about different aspect of a construct.

Threats to construct validity, defined as erroneous inferences from the particular evaluation study to the higher level abstract concept, must be considered. Threats can occur if there is a mismatch between the higher-level concept of interest (e.g., interdisciplinary collaboration) and how the evaluator has operationalized the concept for purpose of the evaluation. It can also occur if irrelevant evidence is collected and included in the evaluation process. Although the evidence may be accurate, it is irrelevant to the focus of the evaluation. Other forms of threats to construct validity include evaluator bias and participant bias, both of which were discussed earlier in this chapter. In thinking about validity, it is never either a present or not present consideration; validity is always a determination of to what degree something is valid.

Contextual and Environmental Dimension of Evidence

In conducting any evaluation, the context and local environment in which the evaluation takes place is important. Stetler (2003) described this evidence source as "internal evidence," which she reports comes primarily from systematically but locally collected information including data from local performance, planning, quality, and outcomes; knowledge about the culture of the organization and the individuals in it; and local and national policy. The focus of the evaluation, regardless if an organization, a group, or an individual is being evaluated, has to be appreciated within the context of the environment in which it operates. There may be special contextual and environmental characteristics unique to the focus of the evaluation that must be taken into consideration. For example, if an evaluator is assisting an organization to determine its readiness to apply for the Magnet Recognition Program offered by the American Nurses Credentialing Center (ANCC), the mission, size, and community in which the organization is located should be considered. A 75-bed, acute care facility located in a rural setting may not have the infrastructure to meet the research expectations of the Magnet criteria. Such a facility may be better positioned to apply for the Pathway to Excellence Program also administered by ANCC with criteria that focuses on use of evidence-based practice rather than generation of new knowledge.

Quality of Evidence

An important distinction is made between strength of evidence systems and evidence hierarchies. Evidence hierarchies focus on the study design, with systematic reviews of randomized controlled trials and individual randomized controlled trials positioned at the highest level. By comparison, strength of evidence systems incorporate not only study design, but also other components such as presence or absence of bias, quality of the evidence, and precision of estimates (Owens et al., 2010). Yet the domains included in the strength of evidence systems are not uniform, thus contributing to the confusion of grading evidence.

Given the movement of the last 20 years to evidence-based practice, several evidence hierarchies have been developed by a number of scholars and organizations to grade scientific evidence according to the quality and strength of the evidence for clinical practice. These hierarchies are specifically designed for scientific evidence most often from publications reporting systematic reviews, randomized controlled trials, quasi-experimental designs, qualitative studies, case reports, and other forms of research. These hierarchies are discussed in Chapter 7. In conducting an evaluation, these evidence hierarchies are not helpful except when a cost effectiveness analysis is conducted because they provide an indicator of effectiveness. They are also helpful when a review of the literature is conducted to determine the state of the science about a particular area of interest addressed through randomized controlled trials or to understand the constructs of interest. Not all questions lend themselves to be investigated through randomized controlled trials. When considering evidence for evaluation, several questions confront the evaluator, such as: what is the strength of the evidence; what is the value of the evidence; how confident are you about the accuracy of the evidence; and can you trust the evidence.

Strength has to do with the capacity to exert influence. In the case of evaluation it is the strength of the evidence that informs the evaluator about the focus of interest. Strong evidence is compelling while weak evidence contributes little or nothing to the evaluation process. Primary evidence is viewed as stronger than secondary evidence. The value of evidence requires judgment by the evaluator and is subject to bias, and often depends upon the purpose for which the evidence is to be used. Purpose helps the evaluator decide what kind of evidence is needed, in what form, and in what amount.

Value of evidence also depends upon the context and environment for which it will be used. Some evidence will be critical based on the context of an evaluation, while other information may be helpful but not critical. Evidence is used to inform decision making and judgment so that the evaluator must determine if the evidence collected is appropriate, useful, credible, accurate, and trustworthy. It may take some investigation to verify that these characteristics of evidence are present. The legitimacy of evidence is always linked to purpose. The evaluator makes judgment on a continuous series of questions throughout the evaluation process. The evaluator's goal is to access the best available evidence possible.

What should the evaluator do if the evidence that he or she planned to collect is not available? There are times when the evaluator does not have access to the evidence that he or he would like to collect. This may be due to evidence not being recorded, the unavailability of an informant, or a limitation of access due to the confidential nature of some information. In such a situation, the evaluator must decide how critical the information is to the evaluation process. Often, some evidence is nice to have but is not critical; in other instances, certain evidence may be critical to the evaluation. The evaluator must determine if there is other available evidence that can substitute or be a proxy for the desired evidence. It may be possible to infer from other pieces of evidence about the area of interest. If the evaluator determines that missing evidence is indeed very important in the evaluation process and is unattainable, then this information should be listed as a limitation of the evaluation.

APNs AND EVALUATION

The interest in evidence by health professionals is related to their need to substantiate the worth of a wide variety of activities and interventions (Pearson, Wiechula, Court, & Lockwood, 2007). The type of evidence sought by the evaluator varies according to the focus of the evaluation, which might be a clinical question, or a question about the nature of an intervention, activity, or focus of interest. The previous discussion provided a background for the evaluation in a generic sense to assist APNs in thinking about evidence. In this final section, the evaluation process focuses on the role of APNs in evaluation.

Role of the APN in Evaluation

APNs often assume responsibility and accountability for evaluation. Evaluation of care for individual patients and populations is an integral part of care. However, APNs may be asked to evaluate any number of practices, interventions, products, programs, and policies either as an individual evaluator or as part of a team of evaluators. Additionally, evaluation in a digital age offers new dimensions to sources of evidence as well as the collection, storage, and organization of evidence. The following provides examples of common types of evaluations that APNs may conduct.

Practices
Clinical practice and the practices or processes involved in providing care are exceedingly complex. For example, the APN may be asked to examine

the hand-off practices by nurses and physicians on a unit or service line. In thinking about this request, the APN considers the many forms of hand-offs in health care. There are nurse-to-nurse hand-offs between shifts, at mealtime, and during transfer to another unit. Physician-to-physician hand-offs occur when a patient is transferred to another unit or another hospital. In a model where physicians are employed by a health care facility to work shifts, such as a hospitalist or resident, there is physician-to-physician hand-off between shifts. The APN evaluating hand-off practices would most likely begin with focusing on the overall evaluation and then conducting a review of the literature to understand the state of the science related to hand-offs. In the process of review, the APN would identify key variables to address and might also find instruments that could be used for collecting and measuring variables of interest. The literature is often a good guide for developing a protocol for the evaluation.

Another example of practice evaluation is one that examines the effectiveness of interdisciplinary teams for their impact on core measures and outcomes. Although it is generally believed that high performance, interdisciplinary teams have better patient and provider outcomes, teasing out the contributions that each team member contributes to outcomes may be difficult to determine. This is an example of a complex evaluation focus that might be conducted by a team that includes an expert consult to guide the process. Sources of evidence might include review of the literature, observation, semi-structured interviews, questionnaires, mining of patient outcome data related to practice processes, cost analyses, and core measures data.

Interventions

Although providers like to think that their practice is evidence-based, it is clear that more than half of what is done in practice has no scientific basis. For example, the nursing practice of turning a patient every 2 hours has no scientific basis. The focus of the evaluation could be to examine the practices of turning patients and the incidence of pressure ulcers in a facility. This information could be of value to a Nursing Practice Committee charged with reviewing patient turning protocols in a long-term care facility. Sources of evidence are similar to practice inquiry and might include review of the literature, observation, semi-structure interviews, questionnaires, mining of patient outcome data related to team performance, cost analyses, and core measures data.

Products

Health care facilities must make decisions on all products, from beds to dressings to educational materials. The decision might be about including new products in a facility or replacing a newer product with an established product. The APN is often asked to evaluate a new product and compare it with current products. The evaluation is not only based on cost, but achievement of stated outcomes, user friendliness, time required by the care provider to use the product, and acceptability by the patient. Because products and equipment are a big part of the operating budget, decisions on product evaluation have ramifications for the cost of health care. Helpful sources of evidence might include the literature on comparative effectiveness with other similar products, interviews with users to determine how it is used, ease of use, reliability, cost, maintenance requirements, contribution to patient care, and return on investment.

Programs

Another type of evaluation that APNs might conduct is that of program evaluation. The program could be a clinical program such as a community-outreach stroke prevention program, an established comprehensive heart failure program within a hospital or system, or an orientation program for newly hired registered nurses on a specialty unit such as an orthopedic service. All programs should first be effective. It is important to understand the purpose of the evaluation. Is the purpose of evaluation for feasibility, impact on a community, or cost? The purpose will determine what evidence will need to be examined. The findings of a program evaluation may lead to a quality improvement project. In the current cost-conscious environment of quality and safety, much emphasis is being placed on comparative effectiveness evaluation to guide decision making. Sources of evidence to evaluate a program might include: the literature; descriptions of characteristics of effective high-performance programs for purposes of focused data collection and comparison; interviews with a broad range of stakeholders including providers, administrators, and recipients about effectiveness and meeting of recipients' needs; patient/client outcome data; cost analysis; analysis on return on investment; projected changes in the program for the future including need for additional resources and cost; and observations of program processes.

Policies

Policies and procedures that guide practice and care must be evaluated and updated on a regular basis to stay current and in compliance with regulatory bodies and professional standards. The APN is often responsible for evaluating and updating policies and procedures as an individual evaluator or as part of a committee or other group advising decision makers. For example, a policy that requires 10 units of continuing education for all nursing staff may be scheduled for review in light of changes make by the state board of nursing for re-licensure. The number of continuing education units may need to be increased because of new mandatory continuing education required by the state. The evaluation process might include current policy, mandatory changes, financial impact on the health care facility to support the continuing education requirements, and methods of communicating the change to staff. Sources of evidence to evaluate policies include a review of the literature, interviews with stakeholders affected by the policy or policies, policy analysis with local and national compliance imperatives, potential consequences of policy change or lack of change, cost implications of policy decisions, and the social environmental impact of the policy. Much of the evidence can be collected from internal sources including people and databases, and then applied to the local and national imperatives and standards required by the organization.

Common Sources of Evidence Used by APNs

Common sources of evidence used by APNs when conducting an evaluation are included in Table 2.3.

TABLE 2.3
Common Sources of Evidence for APNs

Source	Examples
Print and electronic sources including data mining from internal and external databases	Journals, websites, electronic databases, books, survey data, dashboards, minutes of meetings, patient medical records, internally developed databases
Observations	Physical examination, participatory interactions (attending meetings, demonstrations)
Interviews	Individuals, groups
Surveys/instruments	Conducted electronically (e.g., Survey Monkey) or paper format reported as aggregate data
Experiments/comparisons	Use of comparison groups or products
Personal experiences	Composite of clinical, professional, and personal experiences gained in a variety of ways
	Practice knowledge (what is learned in practice)
Reflections	Linking knowledge learned from patient care or other experiences with other forms of knowledge to provide best practice
	Seeing similarities in a new patient situation with previously accumulated knowledge from other cases

In planning any evaluation, regardless if it appears simple or complex, careful attention must be paid to design. Design includes thinking prospectively of all possible factors that could undermine the quality of the evaluation including bias and validity. Although evaluation is generally considered at the end of many processes, it should be integrated early into the planning stage of any new projects. The steps to conducting an evaluation are discussed in Chapter 1.

SUMMARY

Evaluation is based on the collection, organization, and critical review of evidence to make decisions about value. Evidence comes from many sources and is found in many forms. The evaluator must not only understand the overall process of evaluation, but also must be able to identify and collect the necessary evidence. The quality of the evidence must be constantly considered including bias, validity, and reliability of evidence that will lead to the best possible evidence that can be trusted for decision making.

REFERENCES

Ackoff, R. L. (1989). From data to wisdom. *Journal of Applied System Analysis, 16*, 3–9.

American Nurses Association. (2001). *Scope and standards of nursing informatics practice.* Washington, DC: American Nurses Publishing.

Angeles, P. A. (1992). *The HarperCollins dictionary of philosophy* (2nd ed., p. 85). New York, NY: HarperCollins Publishers.

Bellinger, G., Castro, D., & Mills, A. (2004). *Data information, knowledge, and wisdom.* Retrieved from http://www.systems-thinking.org/dikw/dikw.htm.

Benner, P. (1984). *From novice to expert: Excellence and power in clinical nursing practice.* London, England: Addison-Wesley.

Benner, P., & Tanner, C. (1987). Clinical judgment: How expert nurses use intuition. *American Journal of Nursing, 87*(1), 23–31.

Billay, D., Myrick, F., Luhanga, F., & Yonge, O. (2007). A pragmatic view of intuitive knowledge in nursing practice. *Nursing Forum, 42*(3), 147–155.

Blackburn, S. (2008). *Oxford dictionary of philosophy.* New York, NY: Oxford University Press.

Carper, B. (1978). Fundamental patterns of knowing in nursing. *Advances in Nursing Science, 1*(1), 12–23.

Copi, I. M., & Cohen, C. (2009). *Introduction to logic* (13th ed.). Upper Saddle River, NJ: Pearson Prentice Hall.

Dictionary.com Unabridged; based on the Random House Dictionary, Random House, Inc. (2010). Retrieved from http://dictionary.reference.com/browse/evidence-9-24-10

Eraut, M. (1985). Knowledge creation and knowledge use in professional contexts. *Studies in Higher Education, 10*(2), 117–133.

Eraut, M. (2000). Non-formal learning and tacit knowledge in professional work. *British Journal of Educational Psychology, 70,* 113–136.

Fawcett, J., Watson, J., Neuman, B., Hinton-Walker, P., & Fitzpatrick, J. J. (2001). On nursing theories and evidence. *Journal of Nursing Scholarship, 33*(2), 115–119.

Freshwater, D., Taylor, B. J., & Sherwood, G. (Eds.). (2008). *International textbook of reflective practice in nursing.* Oxford, UK: John Wiley & Sons Ltd.

Gallagher, T. K. (1964). *The philosophy of knowledge.* New York: Sheed and Ward.

Goldberg, M. J. (2006). On evidence and evidence-based medicine: Lessons from the philosophy of science. *Social Science & Medicine, 62,* 2621–2632.

Goodman, K. W, (2003). *Ethics and evidence-based medicine: Fallibility and responsibility in clinical science.* Cambridge, UK: Cambridge University Press.

Graves, J. R., & Corcoran, S. (1989). The study of nursing informatics. *IMAGE: Journal of Nursing Scholarship, 21*(4), 227–231.

Guyatt, G., Rennie, D., Meade, M. O., & Cook, D. (2008). *Users' guide to the medical literature* (2nd ed.). New York, NY: McGraw-Hill.

Higgs, J., & Titchen, A. (1995). The nature, generation and verification of knowledge. *Physiotherapy, 81*(9), 521–530.

Husserl, E. (1982). *Ideas pertaining to a pure phenomenology and a phenomenological philosophy: First book: General introduction to a pure phenomenology* (F. Kersten, Trans.). The Hague, Netherlands: Nijoff.

Johns, C., & Freshwater, D. (2005). *Transforming nursing through reflective practice* (2nd ed.). Oxford, UK: Blackwell Publishing.

Knowles, E. (Ed.). (1999). *The oxford dictionary of quotations* (5th ed., p. 396). Oxford, UK: Oxford University Press.

Kuhn, T. (1996). *The structure of scientific revolutions* (3rd ed.). Chicago, IL: University of Chicago Press.

Mantzoukas, S. (2007). A review of evidence-based practice, nursing research, and reflection: Leveling the hierarchy. *Journal of Clinical Nursing, 17*(2), 214–223.

Melnyk, B., & Fineout-Overholt, E. (2011). *Evidence-based practice in nursing and healthcare* (2nd ed.). Philadelphia, PA: Lippincott Williams & Wilkins.

Mitchell, G. J. (1994). Intuitive knowing: Exposing a myth in theory development. *Nursing Science Quarterly, 7*(1), 2–3.

Owens, D. K., Lohr, K. N., Atkins, D., Treadwell, J. R., Reston, J. T., Bass, E. B., ... Helfand, M. (2010). AHRQ series paper 5: Grading the strength of a body of evidence when comparing medical interventions–Agency for Healthcare Research and Quality and the Effective Health-Care Program. *Journal of Clinical Epidemiology, 63,* 513–523.

Parse, R. R. (1981). *Man-lining-health: A theory of nursing.* New York, NY: John Wiley & Sons.

Parse, R. R. (1992). Human becoming: Parse's theory of nursing. *Nursing Science Quarterly, 5*(1), 35–42.

Pearsall, J., & Trumble, B. (Eds.). (1995) *The oxford encyclopedia dictionary* (2nd ed.). New York, NY: Oxford University Press.

Pearson, A., Wiechula, R., Court, A., & Lockwood, C. (2005). The JBI model of evidence-based healthcare. *International Journal of Evidence-Based Healthcare, 3,* 207–215.

Pearson, A., Wiechula, R., Court, A., & Lockwood, C. (2007). A re-consideration of what constitutes "evidence" in the health care professions. *Nursing Science Quarterly, 20*(1), 85–88.

Polit, D. F., & Beck, C. T. (2008). *Nursing research: Generating and assessing evidence for nursing practice* (8th ed.). Philadelphia, PA: Wolters Kluwer/Lippincott Williams & Wilkins.

Rycroft-Malone, J., Seers, K., Titchen, A., Harvey, G., Kitson, A., & McCormack, B. (2004, July). What counts as evidence in evidence-based practice? *Journal of Advanced Nursing, 47*(1), 81–90.

Schon, D. (1983). *The reflective practitioner*. London, UK: Temple Smith.

Schon, D. (1987). *Educating the reflective practitioner*. San Francisco, CA: Jossey-Bass.

Shadish, W. R., Cook, T. D., & Campbell, D. T. (2002). *Experimental and quasi-experimental designs for generalized causal inference*. Boston, MA: Houghton Mifflin.

Stetler, C. (2003). The role of the organization in translating research into evidence-based practice. *Outcomes Management for Nursing Practice, 7*(3), 97–103.

Streubert-Speziale, H. J., & Carpenter, D. R. (2003). *Qualitative research in nursing: Advancing the humanistic imperative* (2nd ed.). Philadelphia, PA: Lippincott.

University of Maryland Libraries. (2006). *Primary, secondary, and tertiary sources.* Retrieved from http://www.lib.imd.edu/guides/promary-sources.html

White, J. (1995). Patterns of knowing: Review, critique, and update. *Advances in Nursing Science, 17*(4), 73–86.

THREE

Conceptual Models for Evaluation in Advanced Nursing Practice

Christine A. Brosnan

"Do not go where the path may lead, go instead where there is no path and leave a trail."

Ralph Waldo Emerson

INTRODUCTION

Evaluation is an essential step in the nursing process. Nurses in undergraduate and graduate programs are taught to assess patient needs, diagnose patient problems, plan for the care of patients, implement that plan of care and then evaluate the results of the care provided (Potter & Perry, 2009). Following the mandate of *The Essentials of Master's Education in Nursing* (American Association of Colleges of Nursing [AACN], 2011) and *The Essentials of Doctoral Education for Advanced Nursing Practice* (AACN, 2006), graduate education programs expanded curriculum content related to evaluation. As a result, practitioners should be able to engage more fully in quality assurance and other evaluation activities. Early evaluations focused primarily on comparing the value of advanced practice nursing to medical care (Kleinpell, 2009). Today, as health professionals and patients become more comfortable with the advanced practice role, the scope and depth of evaluations are increasing.

While nursing is an essential component of the health care delivery system, other providers also directly impact health status. Medicine, respiratory therapy, physical therapy, and pharmacy are some examples of disciplines to include in a comprehensive evaluation of patient care. The definition of *patient/client* and the focus of an evaluation have also expanded in advanced practice. As noted in Chapter 1, *patient* may now be defined as an individual, a group, a community, or a population affected by the health care activity being evaluated. The evaluation may not focus solely on direct patient care. The APN may be asked to participate in the evaluation of technologies, programs, guidelines/protocols, information systems, health education programs and policies. Depending upon knowledge, experience, and skill set, the nurse may be a leader or a member of an interdisciplinary evaluation team.

The conceptual foundation that supports the expanded scope of evaluation is interdisciplinary and continues to evolve. This chapter reviews major theories and concepts that form the basis of evaluation in advanced practice nursing. Donabedian's conceptual model, introduced in the first chapter, is discussed in more depth. Not only is his model directly used in health care evaluation, but his concepts have also been adapted for use in the development of alternative evaluation models.

The Effectiveness-Efficiency-Equity conceptual framework developed by Aday, Begley, Lairson, and Balkrishnan (2004) is presented. Aday's framework is eclectic, integrating some of Donabedian's concepts with constructs from epidemiology, sociology, ethics, economics, and the behavioral sciences. It has application across a variety of settings and types of perspectives. It is particularly relevant to the evaluation of policies affecting populations.

The chapter discusses the development and application of logic models. These models provide a blueprint to guide the evaluation process and illustrate how the components of the evaluation process relate to each other. Logic models are quite popular today, particularly among funding agencies.

The conceptual framework, Monitoring and Evaluating Health Systems Strengthening, developed by the World Health Organization (WHO) and other international organizations, is also described (Boerma et al., 2009). The model is particularly useful for the evaluation of very large health care systems, such as those at the national level.

CONCEPTUAL MODEL: S-P-O MODEL

Donabedian's contribution to developing a systematic and objective method of ensuring the quality of health care evolved over four decades beginning in 1966 when he first introduced his framework for evaluating quality in health care. He observed that quality meant different things to different people: "The definition of quality may be almost anything anyone wishes it to be, although it is, ordinarily, a reflection of values and goals current in the medical care system and in the larger society of which it is a part" (Donabedian, 1966, p. 167). He suggested that one could evaluate quality using three approaches individually or in combination: One could focus on the structure of care, on the process of care, or on the outcome of care. Donabedian identified basic problems in successfully conducting systematic and objective evaluations regardless of approach. These include: (a) a lack of valid and reliable measures, (b) the limitations of data sources and standards of measurement, (c) inadequate measurement scales, and (d) difficulty in establishing the link among each of the three approaches (structure, process, and outcome). Donabedian spent the rest of his professional career (and his life) examining these concerns and their relevance to improving the health of patients.

Health and Health Care

At the most basic level, health focuses on biophysical status (Donabedian, 1987). Practitioners assess the baseline health status of a patient, diagnose the condition, develop a plan of care, and intervene with evidence-based treatment. Outcome evaluation focuses primarily on the positive or negative changes in health status that result from the treatment provided. For example, in evaluating the outcome of individual care, a practitioner might measure the change in temperature and laboratory values after a patient with the H1N1 influenza is treated appropriately with medication and IV fluids. In evaluating a program, a practitioner may measure the change in the number of cases of H1N1 diagnosed in a community as a result of an immunization program. In evaluating population health, a practitioner may measure the change in the number of deaths caused by H1N1 in a city before and after the availability of immunizations.

An expanded description of health includes a sense of well-being that can be associated with quality of life (Donabedian, 1987, 2003). Determining the effect of an intervention or program on quality of life is challenging. For instance, a pacemaker inserted in the chest of a patient with dementia may improve the patient's health status but may not improve the patient's sense of well-being. Individuals differ and that makes it difficult to define and measure quality of life. Consider two patients who must have a below-the-knee amputation as a result of diabetes mellitus complications. One patient may have strong family and social supports, adapt to the disability and rate the resultant quality of life as good. The other patient may have fewer resources and judge quality of life as poor. Health service researchers have spent decades developing measures that attempt to quantify and standardize the term. Quality of life will be discussed in greater detail in Chapter 4.

Evaluation functions at the macro, meso, and micro levels. Periodically, it is important to examine the totality of care provided by a nation (macro level) or governmental agency (meso level) to meet the health care needs of a population. Care provided to patients and groups of patients at the micro level should be monitored more frequently. If health care at the micro level is found to be less than optimum, practitioners can make appropriate changes that will theoretically impact care at the macro and meso levels. Quality assurance at all three levels provides the most comprehensive analysis (Donabedian, 1987).

APNs frequently participate in monitoring activities and Donabedian's framework provides a method for deciding what indicators to monitor (Donabedian, 2003). Some indicators are externally imposed, such as those required by external organizations and agencies in order to maintain accreditation or to establish a unique status. The Joint Commission, Centers for Medicare and Medicaid Services, and the American Nurses Credentialing Center Magnet Recognition Program are examples of external influences on monitoring health care.

Other quality assurance indicators arise from local institutional concerns. These may focus on specific internal indicators selected either as a result of administrative planning or because an adverse event presents an opportunity for further examination. As an example of administrative planning, the Director of Nursing of a medical clinic establishes an interdisciplinary quality improvement committee to identify problem areas and concerns. The committee requests chart audits and surveys to detect untoward trends that merit further study. The committee reports to the Director that during the past year, the number of diabetic patients returning for periodic eye exams has decreased. The committee recommends that all patients receive letters reminding them about their next scheduled follow-up visit and a brief statement about the importance of eye testing. The committee further suggests that the number of patients returning for follow-up be reanalyzed in one year.

An adverse event or a sudden rise in complaints may trigger monitoring activities. As an example, the Director of Quality Improvement notices a 50% increase in the number of patient complaints related to the timeliness of receiving p.r.n. pain medication. The Director asks the Quality Improvement Committee to examine the problem and report their findings. Chart audits, staffing records, and interviews reveal a problem of nighttime understaffing. The Director of the Quality Improvement Committee forwards the report to the Director of Nursing for feedback and recommendations.

It is not feasible to evaluate all indicators at the same time, therefore priorities must be established. There is no hard and fast rule in setting priorities, but problems that pose a direct risk to patient health should be a primary concern. Practitioners also need to consider the extent of the problem and the feasibility of fixing the problem (Donabedian, 2003).

Defining the Pathways to Quality Assurance: Structure, Process, and Outcome (S-P-O)

At the most basic level quality is an assessment of the "technical performance of individual health care practitioners" (Donabedian, 1987, p. 75). An expanded description provides contextual components of the interaction between patient and practitioner. Contextual components include: patient adherence to practitioner recommendations, the barriers and facilitators to obtaining health, and the hospital or clinic environment.

Donabedian's model lays out three approaches or pathways to evaluating health care: structure, process, and outcome. *Structure* refers to the administrative support provided for quality care and the environment in which health care occurs. Adequacy of supplies and equipment, number and proficiency of health care personnel, the hospital environment, and barriers and facilitators to access are structural components (Donabedian, 1987, 2003). Tarlov et al. (1989) also included patient characteristics like age, comorbidity, risk, and beliefs under the category of structure.

Process comprises practitioner-patient interactions and the practitioners' technical proficiency in their therapeutic relationships with patients. Process measures offer a direct approach to evaluating health care quality because health care that meets best practice standards in a specific time and place is quality care. Inherent in the selection of process criteria is the assumption that a strong link exists between how providers interact with patients and the outcomes of care (Donabedian, 1966, 1978, 2003). The type and number of diagnostic tests ordered, differential diagnoses listed, interpretation of test results, treatment prescribed, and type of patient education are all process characteristics (Donabedian, 2003; Tarlov et al., 1989). Process indicators reflect current standards of practice and, as a result, evolve over time (Larson & Muller, 2002).

Outcomes refer to a measurable change in patient health status that results from health care delivered (Donabedian, 1988, 2003). Measuring outcomes does not provide as direct a path as process in evaluating quality but outcomes are "the ultimate validators of the effectiveness and quality of medical care" (Donabedian, 1966, p. 169). An advantage of outcomes is that they are recognizable to both practitioners and patients. Practitioners can measure the effect of a treatment and patients can report if a treatment made them feel better or worse. Another advantage is that desired outcomes can be standardized across settings. A 10% reduction of nosocomial infections in a hospital is a beneficial outcome that can be compared to other hospitals regardless of geographic location.

Outcomes may be generic or specific to a disease (Donabedian, 2003). Generic outcomes such as mortality and life expectancy are generally influenced by more than disease and reflect the culture and values of family and society. Disease-specific outcomes provide a better link to the quality of health care provided. For example, a practitioner determines that mortality among a group of patients with atherosclerosis is higher than among patients without atherosclerosis (a generic outcome). Unless investigated further, the practitioner cannot conclude that the higher mortality is a direct result of atherosclerosis because it could have been caused by other factors common to the age group at risk for atherosclerosis, such as cancer, accidents, pneumonia, etc. On the other hand, an evaluator might audit clinic records to determine the range of high density lipoproteins (HDL) and low density lipoproteins (LDL) cholesterol values in patients with atherosclerosis and hyperlipidemia (a disease-specific endpoint). Determining that 90% of patients have cholesterol values within a normal range after one year of treatment provides evidence that intervention has been effective in lowering cholesterol.

When we focus on only one path to quality we assume that there is a strong correlation among structure-process-outcome (Donabedian, 1987; Larson & Muller, 2002). If we evaluate only outcome we assume that the change in health status was a result of the structure and/or process of care. For example, a practitioner assumes that a decrease in blood pressure in a hypertensive patient indicates that the treatment prescribed was correct. However, in actuality the patient stopped taking the prescribed medication because of the unpleasant side effects associated with it. The patient's blood pressure decreased when the patient resigned from a stressful job. The practitioner wrongly assumed that there was a link between the medication (process) and improved health status (outcome).

Establishing links among the approaches to quality can be challenging although a valid and reliable link must be demonstrated if the evaluation is to be trusted (Donabedian, 1978). Over time, evaluators have found a stronger correlation between process and outcome indicators than between structure and process or between structure and outcome indicators. This may be due to a lack of research in establishing the effect of structure on quality. It does not mean that structural indicators should be ignored; rather, each approach should be viewed as providing unique and complementary information. Taken together they provide the most comprehensive evaluation of quality care (Donabedian, 1978, 2003).

Criteria and Standards

Criteria, standards, and norms are key components in Donabedian's framework, yet their definition and application often lack clarity and consistency across evaluations (Donabedian, 1981, 1982). Donabedian addressed this problem by comparing and contrasting the terms. He described criterion as "an attribute of structure, process, or outcome that is used to draw an inference about quality" (Donabedian, 2003, p. 60). He defined a standard as a "specified quantitative measure of magnitude or frequency that specifies what is good or less so" (Donabedian, 2003, p. 60). Acting together, criteria and standards are the means by which evaluators actualize the conceptual model of S-P-O.

For example, a structural criterion for providing quality care in a nursing home might be the number of registered nurses who staff the facility; the associated standard might be that the facility will not have less than one registered nurse on each shift (Table 3.1). A process criterion might be the number and percent of patients assessed for decubitus ulcers; the associated standard might be that 100% of patients will be assessed daily for pressure ulcers. An outcome criterion might be the number of patients with decubitus ulcers; the associated standard might be that no patient will develop a pressure ulcer.

TABLE 3.1

Examples of Criteria and Standards

Approach	Criterion	Standard
Structure	RNs staffing a nursing home	No less than one RN on each shift
	Protocol for screening patients with diabetes mellitus	Protocol will include measuring Hgb Ac and blood pressure at each clinic visit
Process	Patients assessed for pressure ulcers	100% of patients will be assessed daily for pressure ulcers
	Patients tested for Hgb A1c and blood pressure	100% of patients will have Hgb A1c and blood pressure measured
Outcomes	Patients diagnosed with pressure ulcers	No patient will develop a pressure ulcer
	Level of Hgb A1c and blood pressure	80% of patients will have Hgb A1c <7 and blood pressure <130/80

Role of Patient/Consumer

Patients play a vital role in evaluating the quality of health care. As one-half of the practitioner-patient dyad, they are well qualified to provide certain input about their care. For example, patients are certainly qualified to rate the "amenities of care" that form the contextual and environmental experience (structure). Was the room clean and odor free? Was the food tasty and delivered promptly? Was parking available and affordable?

Patients provide a unique perspective in rating the technical proficiency and interpersonal skills of their practitioners (process). Did the practitioner explain the problem and interventions clearly? Did the practitioner appear caring? Did the practitioner spend time answering questions? Was the staff pleasant and respectful? Although they may not understand the intricacies of technology, patients do know if a procedure made them feel better or worse (an outcome). Did treatment improve their ability to perform activities of daily living? Did treatment enable them to return to work? (Donabedian, 1980, 1992, 2003).

Evaluators must bear in mind that, for a variety of reasons, patients are not always the best judges of quality. The amenities that please one patient may cause distress in another. For example, one patient's hospital experience may be improved by having a roommate while another patient prefers to be alone. Some patients focus on interpersonal relationships while others are more concerned with technical performance. Expectations of successful outcome may or may not be realistic. Regardless of limitations, patient input is an essential component in determining quality of care (Donabedian, 1987, 1992, 2003; Larson & Muller, 2002).

Application of the S-P-O Conceptual Model

From a practical perspective, the most important attribute of the S-P-O Model is how robust it has proven to be over time. The concepts are so universally accepted that practitioners may assume that the categories of S-P-O have always been part of quality assurance. In fact, the framework has evolved and adapted as practitioners increasingly apply it in innovative and novel ways. Five studies that illustrate how Donabedian's model adapts to a variety of settings and clinical specialties are presented in Table 3.2 and discussed in the following.

Kilbourne, Fullerton, Dausey, Pincus, and Hermann (2010) were concerned that patients with major mental health disorders frequently receive less than optimal care when they are diagnosed with accompanying substance abuse and medical problems. Using Donabedian's model they sought to develop a method to identify S-P-O measures with the goal of improving quality of care. They identified structural measures including the availability of medical care practitioners, practitioners with substance abuse knowledge, readiness of hospital beds for patients with dual diagnoses, and patient compliance with evidence-based treatment protocols. Process measures focused on screening and treatment for substance abuse and diagnosis of problems related to diabetes mellitus and hypertension, co-morbidities common in this patient population. Process measures were linked to outcomes that included patient satisfaction, morbidity, and mortality data. The authors noted that it was not difficult to obtain data about structural measures because there was no need to rely on patient records, but it was difficult to establish the link between structure and process and between structure and outcome. They determined that the comprehensiveness of the S-P-O Model was an advantage in successfully evaluating care provided to this patient population. They resolved to apply and assess the validity of Donabedian's model in future studies.

Cornwell, Chang, Phillips, and Campbell (2003) sought to apply Donabedian's model to improve quality of care in a Level 1 Trauma Center. They collected data for 2 years and then introduced substantive structural changes designed to provide more comprehensive patient care. Changes included establishing a designated Level 1 Trauma Unit, increasing professional staff, developing guidelines and protocols, and creating programs to support quality assurance efforts. The authors measured the result of the modifications on process and outcome variables over the following 2-year period. Selected process variables included time spent in the trauma unit and length of time ambulances were forced to bypass the unit because of lack of space. Outcome variables included mortality, length of hospital stay, and length of ICU stay. The authors determined that structural changes were linked to improved time to treatment, decreased bypass time, and decreased mortality among head trauma patients.

Chou et al. (2009) noted the growth of genetics in the United States and explored the extent to which genetic services in the United States have maintained quality standards. They applied Donabedian's framework to their systematic review of the literature because of its comprehensiveness and popularity. The authors included 29 structure-related articles, 19 process-related articles, and 7 outcome-related articles. They found Donabedian's model appropriate for this study and for similar quality improvement studies. They recommended that policymakers encourage evidence-based studies that document the quality of genetic services, particularly the links among structure, process, and outcome indicators.

Liebel, Friedman, Watson, and Powers (2009) also applied Donabedian's model to guide a systematic review of the literature. However, they examined the impact of nursing interventions on the health status of disabled elderly patients. Based on inclusion and exclusion criteria, they selected 10 of 125 articles to review. They found it difficult to establish a direct relation between nursing interventions and improved outcome, but it appeared that health status (as measured by disability level) improved when educated and experienced nurses provided comprehensive and coordinated care. Although their focus was different, the conclusions reached by Liebel et al. were similar to Chou et al. They determined that Donabedian's model was valuable, particularly as it provided a comprehensive evaluation of quality and enabled the authors to identify indicators for further study. They also noted that future studies examining the impact of nursing on the quality of health care to disabled elderly patients should collect evidence concerning the link between nursing visits and improved patient outcomes.

The last example applied Donabedian's framework quite differently than the previous studies. In a pilot project, Upenieks and Abelew (2006) used a qualitative design to describe the administrative efforts of two hospitals attempting to develop a "magnet culture." Authors interviewed a total of 24 administrative and staff nurses to gain knowledge about the structural and process changes that accompany the shift from a nonmagnet to a magnet culture. Structural characteristics included an administrative commitment to magnet status as evidenced by the provision of appropriate continuing education offerings, staffing, technological support, and acceptable salaries. Process characteristics included interprofessional governance and collaboration, a focus on evidence-based patient care, and mentoring. The authors concluded that these characteristics are essential to the attainment of magnet status.

Although these examples represent very disparate uses of Donabedian's S-P-O Model, all have in common a precise identification of the aspects of structure, process, or outcome as they relate to the study. In each case, the model facilitates an objective and systematic assessment of health care quality and a direction for future evaluations.

TABLE 3.2

Examples of Evaluative Studies Using Structure-Process-Outcome

Study	Structure	Process	Outcome	Findings/Conclusions
Kilbourne et al. (2010)				
Developed a framework to measure quality of care in patients with mental disorders and comorbidities	Number of general practitioners available Percent of mental health practitioners with knowledge of substance abuse Number of dual-diagnosis beds available Compliance to evidence-based care	Percent of patients receiving recommended screening for lipids and hypertension Percent of patients with diabetes who had annual eye and foot exams Percent of patients with substance use screening Percent of patients receiving substance use care	Percent with acceptable screening results Patient satisfaction Mortality Addiction severity index changes Percent going back to work	Authors plan to apply the framework and evaluate results
Cornwell et al. (2003)				
Modified and evaluated quality of care at a Level 1 Trauma Center based on Donabedian's model	Increased full-time and part-time faculty Established a trauma admit unit Developed protocols and core curriculum for professional staff Developed programs in QA, research, injury prevention, and outreach Obtained state Trauma Level 1 designations	Time in Trauma Department Time to Operating Room Time to ICU Time to Observation Ward Length of bypass time	Mortality Length of hospital stay Length of stay in ICU	Decrease in overall chance of dying Decreased times to transfer patients to Operating Room, ICU and Observation Decrease bypass time Decrease in length of hospital stay Increase in ICU length of stay

Chou et al. (2009)

Systematic review assessed the evidence base of quality in genetic services	Access to care Health information and databases Medical home and service organization Workforce issues Program development	Patient-practitioner relationships Providing, coordinating and managing care Quality assurance methods	Outcomes specific to genetics Outcomes in general Specific and general outcomes	Donabedian's model provided a good framework for evaluating quality of care Identified the need to develop evidence linking the structure and process of genetic services to improved outcomes

Liebel et al. (2009)

Determined the quality of nursing interventions on elderly patients with disabilities	Conceptual framework Education, experience and training Scheduled time, frequency and duration of visits Patient characteristics	Nurse-patient relationship Assessment Care and management Extent of coordinated care	Disability	Difficult to consistently link changes in disability with nursing care Education, experience, and training was associated with improved disability Comprehensive assessment and coordinated care was associated with improved disability

Upenieks and Abelew (2006)

Examined the cultural status of nursing during application for magnet status	Administration's commitment to nursing Staffing and pay Continuing education and clinical ladders Technology support	Interprofessional governance Collaboration among professionals Evidence-based practice Staff education about magnet status Focus on patient care Mentoring	Magnet status	Structural and process factors must be in place to attain magnet status

CONCEPTUAL FRAMEWORK: EFFECTIVENESS-EFFICIENCY-EQUITY

Aday collaborated with economists, physicians, and other health service researchers in developing an integrated and comprehensive framework (Figure 3.1) that evaluates health policies based on three principal criteria: effectiveness, efficiency, and equity (Aday & Andersen, 1974; Aday et al., 2004). The model addresses the interactive nature of policy and health care quality by providing practitioners with methodologies to measure the impact of policy and the skills to influence policy changes. Depending upon the goal, evaluation may be at the micro, meso, or macro level.

In the Effectiveness-Efficiency-Equity framework, health care policies are viewed from the perspective of the practitioner/researcher who seeks to understand the intricacies and variety of policies at the local, state, and federal level (Aday et al., 2004). The practitioner examines the positive and negative ways that policy affects the health status of individuals, communities, and populations; compares and contrasts the impact of alternate health care programs; and offers recommendations to administrators and lawmakers who ultimately make health care policy decisions (Aday & Andersen, 1984; Phillips, Mayer, & Aday, 2000; Quill, Aday, Hacker, & Reagan, 1999).

Aday and colleagues adapted Donabedian's S-P-O Model to categorize the components of their framework and to provide an approach for evaluation (Figure 3.1). The system for delivering health care, the population projected to need health care, and the setting in which the population lives comprise the structure of care. The attained access to health care and the health risks of the patients seeking care comprise the process of care. The health status of individuals and populations comprise the outcome of care. Effectiveness, efficiency, and equity in health care are the criteria on which these outcomes are evaluated.

The authors defined *effectiveness* as "the degree to which improvements in health now attainable, are, in fact, attained" (Aday et al., 2004, p. 57). In analyzing effectiveness, the practitioner includes not only improvements resulting from the health services provided, but also improvements associated with the familial, cultural, and environmental settings. Effectiveness can further be evaluated at the micro (clinical) and macro (population) levels. Clinical effectiveness relates primarily to changes in the health status of individuals through the health care provided. Population effectiveness relates to changes in the overall health status of populations achieved through health care and environmental factors (Aday et al., 2004).

Efficiency refers to both the production and allocation of health care services. Aday et al. (2004, p. 121) refer to production efficiency as "producing a given level of output at a minimum cost." They refer to allocative efficiency as the "attainment of the 'right,' or most valued, mix of outputs" (Aday et al., 2004, p. 121). Efficiency can be viewed from a macro or micro perspective (Aday et al., 2004). The APN will not normally be involved in evaluating efficiency at the macro level, but may be called upon to collaborate with

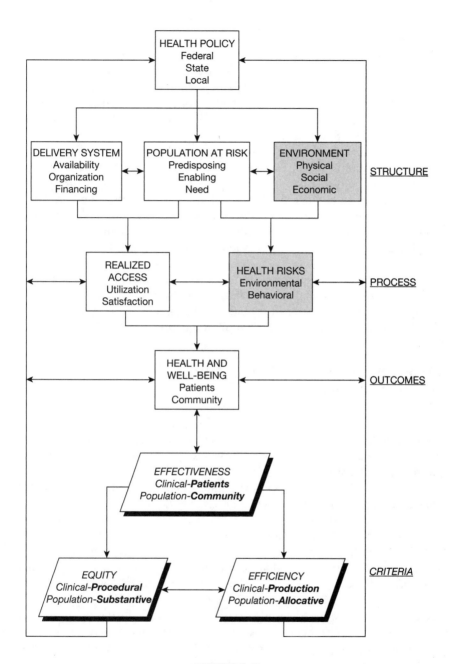

FIGURE 3.1
Framework for applying health services research in evaluating health policy.
Adapted with permission from *Evaluating the health care system* by L. A. Aday,
C. E. Begley, D. R. Lairson, and R. Balkrishnan, 2004,
Chicago: Health Administration Press, p. 14.

other health professionals in conducting micro level evaluations. For example, the practitioner may be asked to determine the best combination of supplies, equipment, and human resources (the inputs) needed to efficiently produce a health care service (Aday et al., 2004). The APN may also be part of a team conducting a cost-effectiveness, cost-benefit, or cost-utility analysis of a technology, service, or program. These evaluation methodologies are commonly used and will be described in Chapter 4.

Equity refers to "maximizing the fairness in the distribution of healthcare (procedural equity) and minimizing the disparities in health across groups (substantive equity)" (Aday et al., 2004, p. 189). Indicators of procedural equity include equality of input into policy decisions, types of facilities and providers available, payment sources, number of services provided, and patient satisfaction. Indicators of disparity in health groups include inequalities with regard to clinical indicators and to population rates of morbidity and mortality. An APN may be called on to collect information about one or more of these indicators in order to determine the equity of current health policies in an agency, community, or population. In evaluating equity, the practitioner examines factors that facilitate and factors that hinder the fair and just distribution of health care across all demographic and clinical groups (Aday et al., 1999, 2004).

Application of the Effectiveness-Efficiency-Equity Conceptual Framework

Three examples in which Aday's conceptual framework was applied are discussed in the following and are presented in Table 3.3. In each case the evaluators sought to inform policy decisions by determining the quality of a health care program.

Begley et al. (2008) examined The Harris County Community Behavioral Health Program, a newly developed program with the goal to improve access to care, improve patient symptoms, and increase provider satisfaction through a combination of behavioral and primary care services. The authors reviewed medical records over an 11-month period to compare utilization of services before and after program initiation. Applying the Behavior and Symptom Identification Scale (BASIS-24) during admission and follow-up visits, they assessed changes in symptoms. Primary care and behavioral providers completed a survey to determine their satisfaction with the program. The authors reported that there was a significant increase in the frequency of visits ($p < .003$) after the program was initiated. They found that patients reported a significant improvement in behavioral symptoms, and that providers were satisfied that the program increased access and quality of care.

Culica and Aday (2008) sought to inform health care policy by comparing utilization, case fatality, and predisposing risk factors in patients admitted to trauma centers versus non-trauma hospitals in Texas during a 2-year period. The authors used a large data base of hospital discharge information that was

TABLE 3.3

Examples of Studies Evaluating Effectiveness, Efficiency, or Equity

Study	Indicators of Quality	Methods	Findings
Begley et al. (2008)			
Evaluated an integrated care program that facilitated access to behavioral and primary care providers in a large publicly funded health care system	Utilization Provider satisfaction Improvement in patient symptoms	Record review comparing utilization before and after program implementation Survey given to providers Compared BASIS-24 at baseline and follow-up	Significant increase in number of visits Program increased utilization, quality of care, time flexibility and interprofessional relations Symptoms significantly improved
Culica and Aday (2008)			
Compared outcomes between trauma centers and non-trauma hospitals	Utilization Case fatality Predisposing risk factors for mortality	Data abstraction from large hospital discharge database	Majority of injured patients (57%) were sent to a trauma center Case fatality higher (3%) in trauma centers compared to non-trauma hospitals (1.25%) Mortality in trauma centers was highest in the young, in males, in ethnic minorities, and in those with no insurance or "other" insurance
Basu et al. (2010)			
Analyzed gender differences in expenditures for treatment of hypertension	Gender disparity Predisposing, enabling, and need factors on expenditures	Data abstraction from the Medical Expenditures Panel Survey	Women generally spent more on treatment of hypertension than men Ratio of women's expenditures compared to men's decreased with age until men spent more than women Predisposing, enabling and need factors did not impact expenditures

obtained from the Texas Health Care Information Council. They reported that the majority of injured patients (57%) were sent to trauma centers, and that case fatality was higher in trauma centers (3% of trauma patients) than in non-trauma hospitals (1.25% of trauma patients). Those who died in trauma centers were more likely to be young, males, members of an ethnic minority, and have either no insurance or "other" insurance, that is, federal programs and insurance methods that were not clearly described. The authors recommended increased collaboration between trauma centers and non-trauma hospitals to decrease the number of less acute patients sent to trauma centers who could be effectively treated at hospitals. They also suggested creating a comprehensive triage system to better coordinate the transfer of patients to each type of facility.

Basu, Franzini, Krueger, and Lairson (2010) analyzed gender disparities related to expenditures for medical care in the treatment of hypertension among adults. They applied the Health Care Use Model (that was integrated into the Framework for Applying Health Services Research in Evaluating Health Policy) to study the influence of population risk factors on gender differences (Aday et al., 2004; Andersen & Aday, 1978). Population risk factors included predisposing factors (age, gender, employment status, education, and race/ethnicity), enabling factors (insurance, economic status, and geographic location) and need factors (comorbidities and current health state). The authors analyzed data from the Medical Expenditures Panel Survey, a national database of health care cost (Agency for Healthcare Research and Quality, 2011). After adjustment for risk variables (predisposing, enabling, and need factors) they determined that over a lifetime, women had significantly greater expenditures than men for treatment of hypertension. Women usually spent more than men when they were young or middle aged and spent less than men as they became older. Men spent less than women when they were young but their expenditures increased with age. The authors concluded that age-related differences in hypertension expenses were not linked to population risk factors. Instead, they suggested that provider attitudes about what is appropriate treatment for males versus females may cause a gender disparity.

LOGIC MODELS

Logic models also have components similar to the S-P-O Model. However, logic models provide a more detailed blueprint of how to plan, implement, and measure performance. Emphasis is placed on first defining endpoints and then deciding on the activities and inputs needed to achieve them. Each component of a logic model is connected to and is a consequence of a prior component. The approach is iterative because activities may be modified if endpoints are not attained. Logic models are frequently used by health professionals from non-profit organizations who are concerned with evaluating mission-motivated rather than profit-motivated endpoints (Chen, 2005; Fitzpatrick, Sanders, & Worthen, 2004). They may be applied at the macro, meso, or micro level.

Logic models are concerned with the inputs (also called resources), activities, and endpoints of a program. Endpoints may be referred to as outputs, outcomes, or impact. Figure 3.2 presents an example of a logic model used by the Centers for Disease Control and Prevention (CDC) Division for Heart Disease and Stroke Prevention. Inputs refer to structural components such as organizational framework, administrative guidelines and protocols, number of health care professionals available, health care environment, and financial resources. Program activities are the processes that take place as a program is implemented. These may include health care interventions, educational activities, or technological services.

Logic models use distinct endpoints defined by scope and time (Fitzpatrick, Sanders, & Worthen, 2004). Although the number of endpoints may vary, there are generally three types of endpoints described in a logic model. The first endpoint is output. *Outputs* are immediate consequences of activities; for example, the number and types of patients receiving a particular health care intervention, the quantity of health education pamphlets delivered to patients, or the total number of hours of screening provided to a community group Outcomes provide evaluators with a specific timeline to measure program performance. They may be short term, mid term, or long term depending upon the project. Outcomes focus on improvements in health status including cognitive, behavioral, and attitudinal change. In some logic models, the term *impacts* is used to represent a long-term endpoint such as a change in policy or population health. There are a number of guidelines available online that facilitate the development of logic models including those developed by the W. K. Kellogg Foundation (2004), and the CDC Division for Heart Disease and Stroke Prevention.

Application of Logic Models

Logic models have been used extensively in a variety of health care programs including a sexual violence prevention program (Hawkins, Clinton-Sherrod, Irvin, Hart, & Russell, 2009), a nurse-managed primary care program (Dykeman,

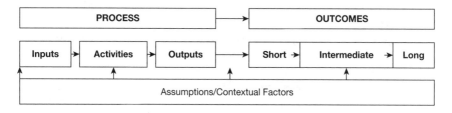

FIGURE 3.2
Layout of a general logic model.
Adapted from *State Heart Disease and Stroke Prevention Program. Evaluation Guide: Developing and Using a Logic Model. Layout of a General Logic Model,* Centers for Disease Control and Prevention Division for Heart Disease and Stroke Prevention, p. 2.

MacIntosh, Seaman, & Davidson, 2003), a statewide heart disease and stroke prevention program (Sitaker, Jernigan, Ladd, & Patanian, 2008), and a teenage pregnancy prevention program (Hulton, 2007). Two examples are provided in the following and in Table 3.4.

Sitaker et al. (2008) discussed the evaluation of a large state program, the goal of which was to assist projects focused on decreasing heart disease and stroke in Washington State. Table 3.4 presents selected input, activity, and outcome indicators that were part of the Washington State Heart Disease and Stroke Prevention Program. Alerting at-risk populations to the signs and symptoms of cardiovascular disease was essential to the mission of the statewide program. The African American Awareness and Screening Project is an example of an activity that received support from the statewide program. As part of the project, health professionals collaborated with barbers and hairstylists in the African American community to inform their clients about cardiovascular disease warning signs and to provide blood pressure

TABLE 3.4

Examples of Studies That Applied the Logic Model

Study	Input	Activities	Outcomes
Sitaker et al. (2008)			
Evaluated a large state program designed to decrease heart disease and stroke	State and federal funding Professional staff Technical help	African American Awareness and Screening Project	*Short-term outcome:* Public awareness of signs and symptoms of heart disease and stroke *Medium-term outcome:* Control of blood pressure and cholesterol *Long-term outcome:* Fewer heart disease and stroke events
Hulton (2007)			
Assessed a school-based teenage pregnancy prevention program	Administrative approval Parental endorsement Curricula Program personnel	Meet with school staff to coordinate schedule Collect data from pre/post surveys Implement educational intervention	*Short-term outcome:* Improve decision-making abilities *Medium-term outcome:* Delay the first sexual encounter *Long-term outcome:* Decreased teen pregnancy rate

screening. Patrons with increased blood pressure were encouraged to seek health care. The authors determined that the logic model allowed them to view this particular project within the context of the overall goals of the program. They were better able to examine the benefits and limitations in a systematic manner and determine the direction of future activities.

In another example, Hulton (2007) used a logic model to evaluate a school-based teenage pregnancy prevention program implemented in a rural community in the northeastern United States. The goal of the program was a decline in adolescent pregnancy in the target population. Collaboration with all stakeholders was considered crucial to the success of the project. Examples of input indicators included administrative approval, parental endorsement, development of suitable curricula based on community values, and expertise of personnel conducting the program. Examples of activities were coordinating program schedules with school staff, collecting survey data before and after the program, and implementing the educational component of a pregnancy prevention program. A desired *short-term outcome* was to improve the students' ability to make good decisions and a *mid-term outcome* was to delay the first sexual event.

Hulton found no significant outcome differences overall between the student group who attended the program and a control group who did not. However, there was a gender difference. Compared to girls who did not attend the program, girls who attended the program were more likely to respond positively about self-efficacy and delaying sex until marriage. Boys who attended the program and boys who did not attend had similar responses. Based on the findings, the author determined that the program was a partial success. The author concluded that the model helped all program stakeholders to work together in establishing and maintaining the systematic tracking of input, activity, and outcome indicators. The model led to increased collaboration and communication among team members and provided direction for making improvements to the program through the development of more targeted activities for boys.

CONCEPTUAL FRAMEWORK: MONITORING AND EVALUATION OF HEALTH SYSTEMS STRENGTHENING

National leaders have long recognized the need to measure the health status of citizens and the benefit of comparing standard health outcomes in one nation to those of other nations. The framework for Monitoring and Evaluation Health Systems Strengthening was developed in response to this need through the collaborative efforts of several international organizations including the World Health Organization (WHO), the World Bank, the Global Alliance for Vaccines and Immunisation (GAVI), and the Global Fund (Boerma et al., 2009). This macro-level framework shares components with the basic logic model described previously. It also provides guidelines for standardizing terms, indicators, and methods with the goal of improving the quality and comprehensiveness of health care evaluation within individual countries and across countries. Although it is recommended for use at the national level, the framework would also be suitable to use at a regional or state level.

The Monitoring and Evaluation (M&E) Framework (Figure 3.3) consists of four main indicator domains: inputs and processes, outputs, outcomes, and impact. The inputs and processes domains contain governance, health financing, infrastructure, workforce, and supplies. The outputs domain contains services readiness and access, and intervention quality, safety, and efficiency. The outcomes domain contains coverage of interventions and risk behaviors and factors. The impact domain contains improved health outcomes and equity, social and financial risk protection, and responsiveness.

An important component of the M&E Framework is the use of valid and reliable core indicators across the domains. The authors recommended that evaluators not only develop indicators relevant to their own target population, but also avail themselves of internationally accepted indicators when appropriate. As in every evaluation, sources for data collection should be relevant and feasible. Such sources include but are not limited to surveys, clinical trials, large national databases, registries, and hospital records. Once obtained, data are analyzed using a variety of statistical tests. Results are first reported to

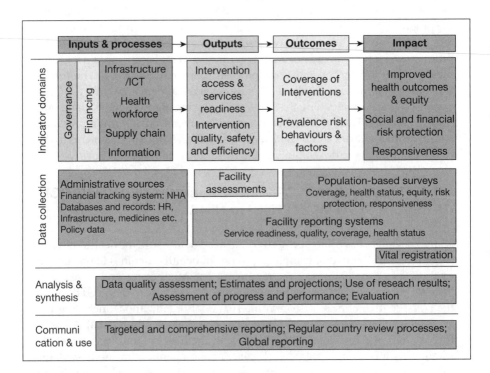

FIGURE 3.3

Monitoring and evaluation of health systems reform/strengthening.

Adapted with permission from *The Monitoring and Evaluation Framework* by the World Health Organization.

the decision makers who requested the information and then disseminated to a wider audience in the form of papers and publications. The ultimate benefit of many nations using the same framework, definitions, indicators, and methods, and then sharing their results, is an increase in the validity of the findings and a better chance that health care programs will be effective, efficient, and equitable.

As an example, an APN might be a member of an evaluation team that is asked to examine the quality of newborn care in a southwestern region of the United States (Table 3.5). One of the first decisions the team makes is it

TABLE 3.5

An Example of the Framework for Monitoring and Evaluation of Health Systems Strengthening: Indicators and Sources for Evaluating Quality of Newborn Care

Domain	Indicators	Sources
Inputs and processes	1. Expenditures for hospital newborn facilities 2. Number of registered nurses/10,000 population 3. Number of neonatal intensive care units per 10,000 population 4. Average cost for oxygen and suction catheters	1. National Health Databases 2. National Nurse Registries 3. Hospital surveys 4. Hospital surveys and facility assessment
Outputs	1. Utilization of registered nurses 2. Geographic location of newborn facilities in relation to population 3. Neonatal case fatality	1. Survey 2. Survey 3. Hospital records and national databases
Outcomes	1. Neonatal after care home coverage 2. Immunization coverage 3. Newborn screening for hearing coverage 4. Breastfeeding for 6 months	1. Survey 2. Medical records 3. National registries 4. Medical records
Impact	1. Child mortality (under 5 years) 2. Hearing disabilities diagnosed in children under 5 years	1. Vital statistics 2. Survey and medical records

to choose indicators and sources to evaluate the four domains (inputs and processes, outputs, outcomes, and impact). Under the domain of inputs and processes, indicators might include hospital expenditures (health financing), registered nurses (workforce), neonatal intensive care units (infrastructure), and average cost for oxygen and suction catheters (supplies). National health databases, registries, surveys, and assessments of clinical and hospital facilities are good sources for these data.

Under the output domain, indicators might include utilization of registered nurses (service readiness), location of facilities (access), and neonatal case fatality (quality and safety). Surveys, registries, hospital records, and national databases are generally used as sources for these types of indicators. Under outcomes domain, indicators might include use of after-care home coverage, immunization coverage, and newborn screening for hearing coverage (coverage of interventions) and breastfeeding for 6 months (risk factors and behaviors). Data could be collected through surveys and medical record review. Impact indicators include child mortality and hearing disabilities diagnosed. Information related to these impact indicators might be obtained from vital statistics, surveys, and health records.

SUMMARY

This chapter explored four conceptual models that have proven valuable in the appraisal of health care quality. The models provide the APN with a framework to systematically and objectively examine interventions, programs, policies, and technologies that affect individuals, groups, and populations.

Donabedian's S-P-O Model is used extensively and adapts to a variety of settings as illustrated in the examples described in the chapter. The Effectiveness-Efficiency-Equity Model developed by Aday and colleagues is particularly useful in obtaining information for the purpose of informing policy decisions. Logic models are widely used in the evaluation of health care programs, and guide the evaluator in determining a program's effectiveness and provide direction in modifying activities. The M&E Framework is suitable for macro-level evaluation of health care quality.

As a member of an evaluation team, an APN will select the model that is most analogous to the purpose of the evaluation. Once the model is chosen, the team must address the challenges inherent in conducting evaluations. Methodological challenges involve selecting valid and reliable measures, establishing associations between the components of the model, and determining the most relevant data sources, data collection methods, and types of analyses. After the results of the evaluation are determined, the team should decide on an appropriate way to report not only the strengths and weaknesses of the intervention, but also the strengths and weaknesses of the evaluation itself. Each of the four models described in the chapter will facilitate a comprehensive and effective evaluation.

REFERENCES

Aday, L. A., & Andersen, R. (1974, Fall). A framework for the study of access to medical care. *Health Services Research, 9*(3), 208–220.

Aday, L. A., & Andersen, R. (1984). The national profile of access to medical care: Where do we stand? *AJPH, 74*(12), 1331–1339.

Aday, L. A., Begley, C. E., Lairson, D. R., & Balkrishnan, R. (2004). *Evaluating the healthcare system* (3rd ed.). Chicago, IL: Health Administration Press.

Aday, L. A., Begley, C. E., Lairson, D. R., Slater, C. H., Richard, A. J., & Menloya, I. D. (1999). A framework for assessing the effectiveness, efficiency, and equity of behavioral healthcare. *American Journal of Managed Care, 5*, SP25–SP44.

Agency for Healthcare Research and Quality. (2011). *Medical Expenditure Panel Survey.* Retrieved from http://www.meps.ahrq.bov/mepsweb/about_meps/survey_back.jsp, 3/12/11

American Association of Colleges of Nursing. (2006). *The essentials of doctoral education for advanced nursing practice.* Washington, DC: Author.

American Association of Colleges of Nursing. (2011). *The essentials of master's education in nursing.* Washington, DC: Author.

Andersen, R., & Aday, L. A. (1978). Access to medical care in the U.S.: Realized and potential. *Medical Care, 16*, 533–546.

Basu, R., Franzini, L., Krueger, P. M., & Lairson, D. R. (2010). Gender disparities in medical expenditures attributable to hypertension in the United States. *Women's Health Issues, 20*, 114–125.

Begley, C. E., Hickey, J. S., Ostermeyer, B., Teske, L. A., Vu, T., Wolf, J., … Rowan, P. J. (2008). Integrating behavioral health and primary care: The harris county community behavioral health program. *Psychiatric Services, 59*(4), 356–358.

Boerma, T., Abou-Zahr, C., Bos, E., Hansen, P., Addai, E., & Low-Beer, D. (2009, November). *Monitoring and evaluation of health systems strengthening.* Geneva, Switzerland: World Health Organization.

Centers for Disease Control and Prevention Division for Heart Disease and Stroke Prevention. (2011). *State heart disease and stroke prevention program. evaluation guide: Developing and using a logic model.* Retrieved from http://www.cdc.gov/DHDSP/index.htm.

Chen, H. T. (2005). *Practical program evlaluation.* Thousand Oaks, CA: Sage Publications, Inc.

Chou, A. F., Norris, A. I., Williamson, L., Garcia, K., Baysinger, J., & Mulvihill, J. J. (2009). Quality assurance in medical and public health genetics services: A systematic review. *American Journal of Medical Genetics Part C (Seminars in medical Genetics), 151C*, 214–234.

Cornwell, E. E., Chang, D. C., Phillips, J., & Campbell, K. A. (2003). Enhanced trauma program commitment at a Level I Trauma Center. Effect on the process and outcome of care. *Archives of Surgery, 138*, 838–843.

Culica, D., & Aday, L. A. (2008). Factors associated with hospital mortality in traumatic injuries: Incentive for trauma care integration. *Public Health, 122*(3), 285–296.

Donabedian, A. (1966). Evaluating the quality of medical care. *Milbank Memorial Fund Quarterly, 44*(Suppl. 3), 166–206.

Donabedian, A. (1978). The quality of medical care. *Science, 200*(4344), 856–864.

Donabedian, A. (1980). *Explorations in quality assessment and monitoring: Vol. I. The definitions of quality and approaches to its assessment.* Ann Arbor, MI: Health Administration Press.

Donabedian, A. (1981). Criteria, norms and standards of quality: What do they mean? *AJPH, 71*(4), 409–412.

Donabedian, A. (1982). *Explorations in quality assessment and monitoring: Vol. II. The criteria and standards of quality.* Ann Arbor, MI: Health Administration Press.

Donabedian, A. (1987). Commentary on some studies of the quality of care. *Health Care Financing Review/Annual Supplement*, 75–85.

Donabedian, A. (1988). Quality assessment and assurance: Unity of purpose, diversity of means. *Inquiry, 25*, 173–192.

Donabedian, A. (1992). The Lichfield lecture. Quality assurance in health care: Consumers' role. *Quality Health Care, 1*, 247–251.

Donabedian, A. (2003). *An introduction to quality assurance in health care.* New York, NY: Oxford University Press.

Dykeman, M., MacIntosh, J., Seaman, P., & Davidson, P. (2003). Development of a program logic model to measure the processes and outcomes of a nurse-managed community health clinic. *Journal of Professional Nursing, 19*(3), 197–203.

Fitzpatrick, J. A., Sanders, J. R., & Worthen, B. R. (2004). *Program evaluation: Alternative approaches and practical guidelines* (3rd ed.). Boston, MA: Pearson Education, Inc.

Hawkins, S. R., Clinton-Sherrod, A. M., Irvin, N., Hart, L., & Russell, S. J. (2009). Logic models as a tool for sexual violence prevention program development. *Health Promotion Practice, 10*(1), 29S–37S.

Hulton, L. J. (2007). An evaluation of a school-based teenage pregnancy prevention program using a logic model framework. *The Journal of School Nursing, 23*(2), 104–110.

Kilbourne, A. M., Fullerton, C., Dausey, D., Pincus, H. A., & Hermann, R. C. (2010). A framework for measuring quality and promoting accountability across silos: The case of mental disorders and co-occurring conditions. *Quality and Safety in Health Care, 19*, 113–116.

Kleinpell, R. M. (2009). *Outcome assessment in advanced practice nursing.* New York, NY: Springer Publishing Company.

Larson, J. S., & Muller, A. (2002). Managing the quality of health care. *Journal of Health & Human Services Adminiatration, Winter*, 261–280.

Liebel, D. V., Friedman, B., Watson, N. M., & Powers, B. A. (2009). Review of nurse home visiting interventions for community-dwelling older persons with existing disability. *Medical Care Research and Review, 66*(2), 119–146.

Phillips, K. A., Mayer, M. L., & Aday, L. A. (2000). Barriers to care among racial/ethnic groups under managed care. *Health Affairs, 19*(4), 65–75.

Potter, P. A., & Perry, A. G. (2009). *Fundamentals of nursing.* St. Louis, MO: Mosby Elsevier.

Quill, B. E., Aday, L. A., Hacker, C. S., & Reagan, J. K. (1999). Policy incongruence and public health professionals' dissonance: the case of immigrants and welfare policy. *Journal of Immigrant Health, 1*(1), 9–18.

Sitaker, M., Jernigan, J., Ladd, S., & Patanian, M. (2008). Adapting logic models over time: The Washington State Health Disease and Stroke Prevention Program experience. *Preventing Chronic Disease, 5*(2), 1–8.

Tarlov, A. R., Ware, J. E., Greenfield, S., Nelson, E. C., Perrin, E., & Zubkoff, M. (1989). The medical outcomes study. *JAMA, 262*(7), 925–930.

Upenieks, V. V., & Abelew, S. (2006). The magnet designation process. A qualitative approach using Donabedian's conceptual framework. *The Health Care Manager, 25*(3), 243–253.

W. K. Kellogg Foundation. (2004). Logic Model Development Guide. Retrieved from http://ww2.wkkf.org/

FOUR

Economic Evaluation

Christine A. Brosnan and J. Michael Swint

"There can be economy only when there is efficiency."

Benjamin Disraeli

INTRODUCTION

APNs are being encouraged to assume greater responsibility in determining the economic efficiency of health care interventions, programs and delivery systems. The American Association of Colleges of Nursing's (AACN, 2011) *Essentials of Master's Education in Nursing* recommended that APNs "apply business and economic principles and practices. . . ." and "employ knowledge and skills in economics. . . . " The AACN's (2006) *The Essentials of Doctoral Education for Advanced Nursing Practice* directed the APN to " . . . evaluate the cost effectiveness of care and use principles of economics and finance to redesign effective and realistic care delivery strategies . . . [and] design, direct, and evaluate quality improvement methodologies to promote safe, timely, effective, efficient, equitable and patient-centered care."

This chapter discusses the increasing importance of economic evaluation, also known as efficiency evaluation, in the provision of health care (Drummond, Sculpher, Torrance, O'Briend, & Stoddart, 2005). The chapter explores the application of economic principles in comparing health care cost and outcomes at the macroeconomic and microeconomic levels. This chapter also reviews the essential concepts and assumptions that support the economic evaluation of health care interventions and programs. The implications of *utility theory* and its impact on health care decisions are discussed. Approaches to valuing health status, including *quality adjusted life years* (QALYs), are explained.

Key terms that provide the basis for different types of economic evaluation are provided in Table 4.1. The chapter reviews the importance of establishing

TABLE 4.1
Definition of Economic Terms

Term	Definition
Charge	The amount of money an institution bills for an item or service (Finkler, 1982)
Cost	The amount of resources used to produce an item or service (Finkler, 1982)
Cost-benefit analysis (CBA)	A comparison evaluation of two or more interventions in which costs and endpoints are calculated in dollars. (Drummond et al., 2005; Torrance et al., 1996)
Cost-effectiveness analysis (CEA)	A comparison evaluation of two or more interventions in which costs are calculated in dollars and endpoints are calculated in health related units (Drummond et al., 2005; Garber et al., 1996)
Cost-utility analysis (CUA)	A comparison evaluation of two or more interventions in which costs are calculated in dollars and endpoints are calculated in quality of life units (Drummond et al., 2005; Torrance et al., 1996)
Direct cost	The money paid for health care (Luce, Manning, Siegel & Lipscomb, 1996)
Discounting	An analyst calculates the current value of future costs and applies that rate to the results of the cost analysis (Muennig, 2008)
Incremental cost	The extra cost and outcome produced by the intervention of interest vs. an alternative intervention or no intervention at all (Drummond, 2005)
Opportunity cost	Represents the money that is spent on one health care intervention that will not be available to pay for a more beneficial alternative intervention (Russell et al., 1996)
Sensitivity analysis	A comparison of a range of costs and endpoints calculated because methods used in the economic analysis were not exact (Manning, Fryback, & Weinstein, 1996; Weinstein et al., 1996)
Perspective	A point of view that reflects the scope of economic responsibility and benefits; establishes the extent of cost and endpoint data that must be collected (Russell et al., 1996)
Quality adjusted life year (QALY)	An endpoint that combines the probability of quantity of life and quality of life years (Drummond, 2005)
Utility	The preference that individuals have for a specific endpoint(s) (Drummond, 2005)

a *perspective* when planning an economic evaluation and discusses the need to *discount* costs and outcomes that occur in the future. The chapter explains the distinction between *costs* and *charges*, and explains why the addition of a *sensitivity analysis* is generally recommended after the results of an efficiency analysis are determined.

This chapter familiarizes the APN with frequently used methods of evaluating health care outcomes along with examples of their application. The role of the APN in applying and participating in economic evaluations is discussed. The chapter presents a guide for critiquing economic evaluations (Exhibit 4.1). A case study is provided at the end of the chapter (Box 4.1).

VALUING HEALTH STATUS

There are basic items that we all value and for which we are generally willing to pay. These items include shelter, food, clothing, and health care. How much each person is willing to pay depends not only upon the resources available,

---

EXHIBIT 4.1
A Guide For Evaluating Economic Studies

1. Was a well-defined question posed in answerable form?

2. Was a comprehensive description of the competing alternatives given? (that is, can you tell who did what to whom, where, and how often?)

3. Was the effectiveness of the programs or services established?

4. Were all the important and relevant costs and consequences for each alternative identified?

5. Were costs and consequences measured accurately in appropriate physical units (e.g., hours of nursing time, number of physician visits, lost work days, gained life years)?

6. Were costs and consequences valued credibly?

7. Were costs and consequences adjusted for differential timing?

8. Was an incremental analysis of costs and consequences of alternatives performed?

9. Was allowance made for uncertainty in the estimates of costs and consequences?

10. Did the presentation and discussion of study results include all issues of concern to users?

From Drummond, M. F., Sculpher, M. J., Torrance, G. W., O'Brien, B. J., & Stoddart, G. L. (2005). *Methods for the economic evaluation of health care programmes* (pp. 28–29). Oxford: Oxford University Press.

but also on the value that is attached to a specific item. One person may spend 10% of the family budget on clothing leaving 90% available for other necessities. Another person may feel compelled to spend 30% on clothing leaving 70% available for necessities. People recognize that their budgets are limited and so they must prioritize their needs, determine their expenses, and adjust their allocations. There is always the risk that those spending 30% on clothing will wind up looking worse than those spending 10%, but that is the chance that they are willing to take. Economists refer to the preference that people have for a particular endpoint or endpoints as their *utility* (Drummond et al., 2005).

Individuals also value health status and are willing to pay for staying healthy and, if they are sick, to pay for effective treatment. However, the path to obtaining preferred health outcomes is not as straightforward as it is for other preferences. Treatment A may be much more costly than Treatment B and the effectiveness of each may not be clear. Even if Treatment A has been shown to be more effective than Treatment B, some individuals may not be able to afford it. Traditionally, society has acknowledged the benefits of a healthy population and has tried to provide essential health care services for those who did not have the means to pay for them, although significant inequities in the availability of health care services exist in the United States.

Over time it has become clear that the amount of money available to spend on health care is finite, and that spiraling costs pose a threat to society. Hiatt (1975) discussed this problem in the context of a "medical commons," the term commons referring to a public area used for grazing cattle (Hardin, 1968). In this example, each farmer wanted to use as much of the commons as possible to feed his herd. Over time farmers kept placing additional cattle onto the commons. The herds grew fat and the farmers prospered, but the unrestricted use eventually resulted in overgrazing and the ultimate destruction of the commons.

Hiatt observed that we inhabit a medical commons in which all individuals want to purchase as much health care as they feel they need. But meeting every individual's perceived need may cost more than society can spend. An unchecked expansion of health spending may eventually mean that society will not be able to provide for other basic items such as education, law enforcement, and defense. Underfunding of these essential items may, in turn, lead to a paradoxical diminishing of our common society's health and welfare (Muennig & Glied, 2010). Some limitation of societal support may be needed, and those purchases with the highest cost and least benefit would be logical targets for elimination. In the last few decades, there have been national initiatives to examine costs associated with health care spending compared to the associated benefits accrued.

A MACROECONOMIC PERSPECTIVE ON COST AND OUTCOME

As part of its mission, the World Health Organization (WHO) collects health data from over 190 countries and uses standard indicators to compare health care costs and outcomes across nations. Costs are expressed as the amount and percent of the Gross Domestic Product (GDP) spent on health care. GDP refers to the final market value of all goods and services produced in a country in a given period of time (World Bank, 2011). National leaders analyze GDP over time and compare their own country's GDP to other countries in order to monitor a country's economic well-being. Health status is measured using standard indicators of mortality and morbidity obtained from national registries. The most recent results, which can be found on the WHO website (http://www.who.int/countries/), provide a rough estimate of the benefits achieved for the amount of resources spent.

A comparison of cost and health status for selected countries is presented in Table 4.2. The cost of health care is expressed in: (a) total international dollars spent for each person and (b) total percent of GDP spent on health care. Purchasing-power parity (PPP) is an approach that states that the exchange rate between one currency and another is in equilibrium when their domestic purchasing powers at that rate of exchange are equivalent (World Bank, 2011). In other words it shows how much of a country's currency is needed in that country to buy what $1 would buy in the United States. Health status is expressed by: (a) probability of dying under 5 years of age per 1000 live births and (b) healthy life expectancy at birth for males and females. In 2008, the United States spent more on health care than each of the other countries listed. With $7,681 in per capita health care spending, the United States was about 2.5 times higher than Japan, Italy, and the United Kingdom, and about twice as high as the expenditures of Canada and France. The percent of GDP spent on health care in the United States (16%) represented a higher percentage on health spending than the other countries. The Center for Medicare and Medicaid Services estimates that by 2015, per capita national health expenditures in the United States will increase to $10,928 and consume 18.9% of the GDP (Center for Medicare and Medicaid Services, 2011).

Despite the effort, U.S. health outcomes did not appear to reflect the generous health expenditures. In 2008, the United States had the highest child mortality (7.8/1000) among the countries listed except for Mexico whose expenditures were $877 per capita. Compared to the United States, life expectancy for males and females was higher in Japan, France, Canada, the United Kingdom, and Switzerland.

These estimates point to the possibility that decision makers in the United States may not always choose the most efficient treatment options. Muennig and Glied (2010) proposed three possible reasons for the discrepancy: (1) Spending on expensive health care interventions may be forcing budgetary constraints in effective public health programs; (2) the increased cost of health care results in an increase in insurance premiums that in turn causes a loss of insurance for those who can no longer afford it; and (3) risks associated with unnecessary interventions may result in an increase in adverse events causing additional morbidity or mortality. In addition, while most economically advanced countries have virtually universal coverage, the United States is an

TABLE 4.2

Cost and Health Status Indicators for Selected Countries

Country Variable	Year	U.S.	Canada	Mexico	Japan	Italy	France	U.K.	Switzerland
Cost									
In international $ per capita, US$ purchasing power parity	2000	4,703	2,519	508	1,969	2,064	2,553	1,837	3,221
	2004	6,196	3,214	689	2,336	2,372	3,121	2,548	3,936
	2008	7,538	4,079	877	2,729	2,870	3,696	3,129	4,627
Percent gross domestic product spent on health care	2000	13.4	8.8	5.1	7.7	8.1	10.1	7.0	10.2
	2004	15.4	9.8	6.0	8.0	8.7	11.0	8.0	11.3
	2008	16.0	10.4	5.9	8.1	9.1	11.2	8.7	10.7
Effect									
Child mortality/ 1000 <5 years*	2000	8.4	6.2	26.0	4.4	5.5	5.3	6.6	5.6
	2004	8.1	6.1	21.3	3.9	4.5	4.8	6.1	5.3
	2008	7.8	6.1	17.5	3.4	4.1	3.9	5.6	4.6
Life expectancy (male/female)	2000	74.1/79.3	76.3/81.7	71.3/76.5	77.7/84.6	76.9/82.8	75.2/82.8	75.5/80.3	77.0/82.8
	2004	74.9/79.9	77.5/82.3	72.0/77.0	78.6/85.6	77.9/83.8	76.7/83.8	76.8/81.0	78.6/83.8
	2008	75.3/80.4	78.3/83.0	72.7/77.5	79.3/86.1	78.7/84.2	77.6/84.3	77.6/81.8	79.8/84.6

From OECD Health data 2010 – selected data. OECD state extracts (http://stats.oecd.org/Index.aspx?DataSetCode=HEALTH).

*Data are available at WHO world health data (http://www.childmortality.org/cmeMain.html).

outlier in this regard. The uninsurance rate in the United States has increased from 14.5% in 1984 to 16.1% in 1995, to an estimated 17.5% in 2009, and evidence indicates that in terms of quality and timeliness, the uninsured do not receive the same standard of care as the insured (Herring, Woolhandler, & Himmelstein, 2008; Institute of Medicine, 2004). Of course we must also recognize that the health of the population is significantly affected by the many social determinants of health; for example, an incidence of smoking that remains too high and the obesity epidemic and resultant increase in the incidence of type 2 diabetes mellitus. As such we have the further issue of deciding how to allocate scarce resources between prevention and cure.

CONCEPTS AND ASSUMPTIONS

The conceptual basis for economic analysis can be found in social welfare theories, particularly those theories dealing with how utilities are allocated in a society (Weinstein & Stason, 1977). As discussed, we assume that good health care is a desired utility, but the resources available for providing health care are limited. How do we as individuals and groups decide what allocation of health resources will most benefit society?

Decisions about funding one health care program over another are made every day. At times decisions are based more on the political environment or popular support and less on the proven benefit of the intervention. Although these are inevitable parts of the decision process, given the scarcity of available resources information from economic evaluations should also be considered by decision makers. The purpose of a health economic evaluation is to collect, analyze, and synthesize objective information about the cost and outcome of health interventions. An intervention may be a treatment, program, or technology (Muennig, 2008). The evaluator compares two or more alternatives, although in some cases the alternative may be the status quo. Evaluations that do not meet the criteria of comparing both cost and outcomes and comparing two or more interventions are called partial evaluations.

It seems obvious that determining the efficiency of an unsuccessful intervention is nonsensical, but it is worth stating again that an intervention must be effective to be cost effective. "If something is not worth doing, it is not worth doing well!" (Drummond et al., 2005, p. 31). Unnecessary or harmful health care not only wastes money and places patients at risk, but it also deprives patients of receiving effective health care because of limited resources.

Opportunity cost represents the benefits foregone when using resources for one health care intervention instead of an alternative intervention (Russell, Siegel et al., 1996). For instance, in considering effective but mutually exclusive interventions (due to budget limitations), the opportunity costs of investing in tuberculosis control instead of investing in diabetes control are the benefits of improved diabetes control that are foregone.

A related concern is that an economic analysis may be viewed as a way to find out how much money a hospital or clinic can make from an intervention. For example, a hospital administrator asks how long a new piece of equipment will take to pay for itself before making a profit. While it is important that hospitals make a profit (as in "No margin, no mission"), the primary focus of an economic analysis is to determine the most efficient way to improve a *patient's health status*, not a *hospital's financial health status* (Porter, 2010).

Establishing the effectiveness of interventions has always presented a challenge to practitioners and researchers (Brook & Lohr, 1985; Buerhaus, 1998; Williamson, 1978). One challenge has been the compatibility of research design and economic analysis. Traditionally, evaluators have relied on randomized controlled trials (RCTs), prospective trials, cohort studies, modeling, and meta-analyses to compare the benefits among alternate interventions (Torrance, Siegel, & Luce, 1996). Each of these research designs has strengths and limitations. The gold standard of cost-effectiveness studies has been an economic analysis alongside a RCT (Drummond et al., 2005). However, experts caution that the economic results might not be practical because the findings obtained under the ideal conditions of an RCT (the efficacy of an intervention) do not represent the findings obtained under real-world conditions (the effectiveness of an intervention). They also suggest that in many cases the results of an RCT are not generalizable (Adams, McCall, Gray, Orza, & Chalmers, 1992; Drummond et al., 2005). Muennig (2008) has recommended applying the standards as described in the levels of evidence when evaluating the quality of studies. (The levels of evidence will be discussed in Chapter 7.) Regardless of flaws, using a systematic and objective method to establish the change in health status is preferable to intuition, guesswork, or no method at all.

A GENERAL DESCRIPTION OF ECONOMIC EVALUATION

There are three types of comparative economic evaluations discussed in this chapter: cost-effectiveness analysis (CEA), cost-utility analysis (CUA), and cost-benefit analysis (CBA). They each represent a full analysis in that the evaluator is describing, measuring, and valuing the costs and outcomes of two or more alternative interventions (Drummond et al., 2005).

Typically, the results of an economic analysis have been presented as a ratio with cost in the numerator and outcome in the denominator. We will discuss some recent modification to this. A practitioner will not only want to know the cost and outcome of an intervention, but also the *incremental cost* and *incremental outcome* of an intervention when compared to one or more interventions. In this context, incremental findings refer to the alteration in cost and outcome produced by the intervention of interest versus the alternative

(Drummond et al., 2005). The findings can be represented in the following ratio adapted from Muennig (2008):

$$\frac{\text{Cost of intervention A } - \text{ Cost of intervention B}}{\text{Outcome of intervention A} - \text{Outcome of intervention B}} \quad \text{(Formula 4.1)}$$

A *cost-effectiveness analysis (CEA)* is a comparative evaluation of two or more interventions in which costs are calculated in dollars (or the local currency) and endpoints are calculated in health related units. The health related units may focus on outcomes such as lives saved or years of living saved, or they may focus on clinical indicators achieved, such as a decrease in blood pressure or cholesterol increments (Drummond et al., 2005; Garber, Weinstein, Torrance, & Kamlet, 1996). The results are given in a ratio with costs in the numerator and health related units in the denominator (Table 4.1). A *cost-utility analysis (CUA)* is a comparative evaluation of two or more interventions in which costs are calculated in dollars (or the local currency) and endpoints are calculated in quality of life units (Drummond et al., 2005; Torrance et al., 1996). Whereas a CEA looks at objective health-related outcomes, in a CUA patients or other affected individuals are asked how they value the outcomes that were or might be achieved. It is an attempt to incorporate the values of the patient (or potential patient) in the decision-making calculus. A *cost-benefit analysis (CBA)* is a comparative evaluation of two or more interventions in which the costs and endpoints are calculated in dollars (or the local currency) (Drummond et al., 2005; Torrance et al., 1996). The results are given in a ratio or as dollars saved or lost. A CBA allows the comparison of investments across alternative interventions (e.g., tuberculosis versus diabetes), whereas a CEA does not. These three types of analyses are comparative evaluations in that all measure costs the same way, but measure and value outcomes differently. Each method provides a unique type of information that may be useful in helping to answer different questions. Occasionally, alternative interventions are evaluated using all three methods simultaneously.

Sometimes an analyst will choose to conduct a partial evaluation instead of a full comparative evaluation. There are two types of partial evaluations. In the first type, an evaluator describes the cost and/or outcomes of an intervention without a comparison (a cost description, an outcome description, or a cost-outcome description). In the second type, an evaluator compares only the costs of two or more alternatives or only the outcomes of two or more alternatives (Drummond et al., 2005).

Before conducting an economic evaluation, an analyst must first decide on the *perspective* of the analysis. Perspective reflects the scope of economic responsibility for costs and outcomes, and it establishes the extent of cost and endpoint information that must be collected (Russell, Gold, Siegel, Daniels, & Weinstein, 1996; Russell, Siegel et al., 1996). For example, a practitioner who conducted an annual diabetes mellitus screening program for a local health clinic may want to determine the cost and outcomes of the intervention from the perspective of the clinic. Cost information would be limited to clinic expenses and outcomes would be limited to the consequences of the program to the clinic population. On the other hand, a practitioner who conducted a state screening program for lead poisoning in children would take a broader, state-level perspective. The collection of cost information would expand to include societal costs at the state level, which might consist of the cost of blood collection, testing the blood, following up abnormal blood tests, making a diagnosis, and treatment. Outcomes would expand to include the benefits and risks (if any) of the state screening program on the population of the state. If the perspective of an analysis is not specified, economists use the national societal perspective as the default perspective.

Once the perspective of an analysis has been established the evaluator can begin to collect *cost* data. The evaluator must first decide what costs should be described, measured, and valued. The *ingredients approach* is one method used to make this determination (Drummond et al., 2005) in which the cost categories of personnel, supplies and equipment, and overhead comprise the components of the cost analysis. *Cost* represents the amount of resources used to produce an item or service and is usually lower than the amount presented as the charge for an item or unit of service. It is preferable to apply cost whenever possible as it more closely reflects actual resource usage. *Charge* represents the amount of money a patient is billed for an item or service. In a sense, it is the asking price and may be only roughly related to the actual resources used for the item or unit of service. Hospital and clinic bills may contain expenditures not intrinsic to the cost of the intervention that were added to increase profits or to offset expenditures in another area (Finkler, 1982). However, Medicare payments are based on the estimated cost of an item or health service unit. As a consequence, Medicare reimbursement is a good data source for establishing the value of health care interventions (Muennig, 2008).

All direct costs are generally included in a cost analysis. *Direct costs* may be described as the expenditures paid for health care. *Indirect costs*, such as productivity costs to the patient and family, include production losses a patient may experience as a result of treatment, including days away from work and time traveled to and from a clinic or hospital (Luce, Manning, Siegel, & Lipscomb, 1996; Muennig, 2008). They may also include other costs, such as the cost to the patient of hiring a caretaker after discharge. Indirect costs may be particularly important to collect when the evaluation takes a societal perspective. Describing, measuring, and valuing indirect costs can be difficult and problematic. If an evaluator decides that the inclusion of indirect costs is not feasible, the exclusion should be noted in the evaluation report.

The cost of an intervention should be adjusted on the basis of timing differences. The adjustment is made when the cost or consequences of an intervention occur in different time periods. This adjustment process is called *discounting*. It involves calculating the current value of future costs and applying the rate to the results of the cost analysis. The rationale for discounting is in part the perception that money spent today is worth more to individuals than money spent one or more years from now. Currently, suggested discount rates for the United States range from 3% to 5%. It is not uncommon to discount cost at one rate (e.g., 3%) for the base case and to provide lower and higher rates (e.g., 1% and 5%) for alternative estimations. By varying the rates an evaluator hopes to offer a range of probable cost approximations (Lipscomb, Weinstein, & Torrance, 1996; Muennig, 2008; Weinstein, Siegel, Gold, Kamlet, & Russell, 1996). In addition to an adjustment for timing, a cost analysis should indicate the country and year of the currency being used (e.g., 2012 U.S. dollars).

There is no perfect economic evaluation. The results of evaluations are frequently approximations because cost and outcome data are uncertain or limited. The result of an analysis that is likely to be the most accurate estimate is referred to as a base case (Russell, Siegel et al., 1996) Economists then use *sensitivity analysis* to adjust for the imprecision inherent in the process. In a sensitivity analysis the analyst varies significant parameters (e.g., the discount rate) and cost and outcome information to determine how these changes impact the findings of an economic evaluation (Manning, Fryback, & Weinstein, 1996; Weinstein et al., 1996). A sensitivity analysis may indicate that the findings of the evaluation are robust or that one or more components need further investigation.

Two examples of partial evaluations that illustrate the components of an economic evaluation are presented in the following and in Table 4.3. Brosnan et al. (2008) conducted a *cost-outcome description* of a high school screening program to identify adolescents who were overweight or hypertensive (Table 4.3). The 2-year project was sponsored jointly by the school district and a school of nursing as part of an ongoing community partnership. The perspective was the cost to the nursing school and a cross-sectional design was used. Community nursing students screened 2,338 students between the ages of 12 and 19 years. Costs incorporated both capital and operating costs. Capital costs (equipment) included stadiometers for measuring height, measuring tapes, and Spacelab monitors for taking blood pressure readings. Operating costs included personnel and supplies. The salaries of nursing faculty, medical faculty, a statistician, and a program coordinator were calculated into personnel costs based on time spent on the project. The potential cost of having nursing students conduct the screening was not included because the endeavor was an integral part of a service learning project and enabled the students to meet course objectives. Overhead costs were excluded because resources of the school of nursing were not used as the project was conducted in area public schools. Costs were discounted at 1%, 3% (the base case), and 5%. Outcomes were body mass index (BMI) and systolic blood pressure (SBP). The base case cost of the screening program was $66,442 (2005 U.S. dollars). A sensitivity analysis was conducted to see how much the total cost of the program would change if a 1% or 5% adjustment was used. The authors concluded that cost varied from a low estimate of $61,417 with a 5% discount rate to a high estimate of $68,429 with a 1% discount rate. Cost per outcome was $72 per student with BMI ≥85th percentile, $107 per student with SBP ≥95th percentile, and $192 per student with BMI ≥85th and SBP ≥95th percentiles. The findings allowed faculty at the school of nursing to estimate the cost of a service learning model.

TABLE 4.3

Examples of Economic Evaluations

Study	Method	Cost	Outcome	Result
Ayadi et al. (2006) calculated cost of a prenatal smoking cessation program	Cost analysis compared three different settings, samples, and implementation methods	Included personnel, supplies, equipment, training, and incentives		Costs ranged from $24–$34 per woman with potential savings of $881 per prenatal woman who quit smoking
Brosnan et al. (2008) determined cost and initial outcomes of screening adolescents for obesity and blood pressure	Cost outcome description	Included personnel, supplies, and equipment	BMI and SBP	$72 per student with BMI ≥85th percentile $107 per student with SBP ≥95th percentile
Graves et al. (2009) evaluated an intensive program to reduce hospital readmission among the elderly versus usual care	Cost utility analysis	Personnel, supplies and material, and cost of hospital or nursing home readmission	Hospital readmission, ER visits, QALYs	Intervention resulted in savings of $333 and 0.118 QALY per person for 24 weeks
Handley et al. (2008) examined an automated telephone self-management support for adults with type 2 diabetes versus usual care	Cost-utility analysis Cost-effectiveness analysis	Personnel, supplies and equipment, and overhead	QALYs 10% increase in disease specific goals	$65,167 per QALY $558 to increase percentage of patients meeting exercise goals

Study	Type of analysis	Costs included	Outcomes measured	Results
Lairson et al. (2008) compared usual care to targeted and tailored reminders for screening	Cost-effectiveness analysis	Personnel, supplies, and overhead	Colorectal screening	Incremental cost was $319 per additional patient screened
Lal et al. (2011) compared stereotactic radiosurgery (SRS) and the SRS plus whole brain radiation therapy (WBRT) treatment arms of a randomized controlled trial of patients being treated for brain metastases	Cost-effectiveness analysis; Cost-utility analysis	Collected data for 7 years, including data for both professional and technical costs	Reported life years saved (LYS) and QALYs; used the time tradeoff method; conducted univariate sensitivity analysis for each probability point estimate	SRS had higher cost than SRS + WBRT ($74,000 vs. $119,000, respectively) 0.60 LYS for WBRT and 1.64 LYS for SRS were reported, resulting in an incremental cost effectiveness ratio of $44,231 per LYS; CUA revealed comparable results, with $41,783 per QALY
McIntosh et al. (2009) evaluated intensive home visits versus standard care to mothers at risk for child neglect or abuse	Cost-effectiveness analysis	Included family and service costs	Maternal sensitivity, infant cooperation and development, environmental support, removal from home	Incremental cost of £3246 per mother compared to standard care. There was a significant increase in maternal sensitivity, infant cooperation, and removal from home if indicated
Siddharthan et al. (2005) examined the VHA for a safe patient handling program versus no program	Cost-benefit analysis	Capital costs, training costs, direct costs associated with treatment and productivity loss	Cost savings related to decreased incidence and severity of injuries	Net annualized benefit of $207,000

Incremental Cost Effectiveness of a Reminder Telephone Call
Program Versus No Program

Program	Cost per Patient	Cost	Incremental Cost	Effect	Incremental Effect: Additional Returned Patients in Method 2 Versus Method 1	Incremental Cost Effectiveness*
1	—	0	—	55	—	—
2	$10	$2,000	$2,000	120	65	$30.77

*The incremental cost per additional patient returned and examined using Method 2 instead of Method 1.

In another example of a partial evaluation, Ayadi et al. (2006) conducted a *cost analysis* to determine the cost and potential savings of a prenatal 5-step smoking cessation program. The 5- to 15-minute program was conducted in three different settings, among different samples, and using different methods of implementation. These included a clinical trial, a telephone quit line, and a managed care agency. The study took a provider perspective and included costs related to personnel, supplies and equipment, training for the counselors, and incentives for the subjects. Centers for Disease Control and Prevention data and software were used to calculate cost savings. Costs were $24 to $34 in the managed care agency, $26 in the clinical trial, and $30 in the telephone quit line intervention. The authors estimated that a potential decrease in neonatal ICU admissions and length of stay could result in a savings of $881(2002 U.S. dollars) per pregnant woman who quit smoking.

TYPES OF ECONOMIC EVALUATION

Cost-Effectiveness Evaluation

As noted, cost-effectiveness analysis (CEA) is a comparative evaluation of two or more interventions in which costs are calculated in dollars and outcomes are calculated in health related units. Cost (the numerator) was discussed in the previous section. This section focuses on health related units (the denominator), which represent the outcome of interventions.

The conceptual models discussed in Chapter 3 provide guidance in selecting appropriate outcome indicators. The primary criterion is that the effectiveness of the intervention has been established. Outcome indicators may be generic or specific to a disease; they may be mid term or long term; they may reference changes in morbidity or mortality. Depending upon the goal, a practitioner may use a number of indicators.

For example, a clinic establishes a program to improve the health status of patients with diabetes mellitus, which is a large segment of the patient population. Intermediate outcomes might be a decrease in blood pressure, decreased hospital admissions, or decreased absence from work. Long-term outcomes may be a decrease in the number of amputations and years of life gained in the patient population. Long-term outcomes are the preferred clinical endpoints but they may be difficult to obtain. When using intermediate endpoints, the analyst should establish the correlation between them and long-term endpoints to the extent possible (Drummond et al., 2005; Torrance et al., 1996).

CEAs are the most frequent type of analysis conducted by nurses (Lämås, Willman, Lindholm, & Jacobsson, 2009) and by other professionals in the health care field. CEAs have several advantages. The information they provide is useful to decision makers who must choose between two or more interventions or programs that have similar endpoints. Because the method has been so widely applied there are many cost-effectiveness studies that nurses will find useful in their practice. Economists have developed guidelines for conducting economic evaluations (Exhibit 4.1) that APNs can use to determine the quality of the studies and the feasibility of applying the results to their practice. A disadvantage is that while CEAs provide information about the change in the quantity of patient health status, they do not address the value to the patient of having achieved the change (Torrance et al., 1996).

Examples of CEAs are discussed in the following and presented in Table 4.3. In the first study, McIntosh, Barlow, Davis, and Stewart-Brown (2009) sought to determine the cost effectiveness of weekly home visits versus standard health and social service care for mothers at risk for child neglect and abuse in England. The design was an economic analysis together with a randomized controlled trial (RCT). The study included 131 women, lasted 18 months, and took a societal perspective. Outcomes were measured using the CARE INDEX, the Brief Infant and Toddler Social and Emotional Assessment, Bayley Scales of Infant Development, and the HOME Inventory. Costs included those incurred by the family, by health, social, and legal services, and by the housing authority. Costs and outcomes were discounted at 3.5% and a sensitivity analysis was conducted. Findings indicated a significant difference between the two groups in maternal sensitivity and infant cooperation. Significantly more infants in the intervention group were removed from the home (4 infants versus 0). The incremental cost of the intervention, £3246 per woman, was significantly higher than standard care (£7120 versus £3874). The study provided decision makers with information that, placed within the setting of the evaluation, was helpful in deciding the value of the program.

In another example, Lairson et al. (2008) compared the cost and effectiveness of usual care to targeted and tailored reminders for colorectal cancer screening during a 2-year period. Targeted reminders consisted of mailed letters containing information and an invitation to be screened. Tailored reminders consisted of additional cues and follow-up telephone calls. The design was an economic analysis together with a randomized controlled trial of 1,546 participants. The perspective was the cost to a clinical agency, which included personnel, supplies and equipment, and overhead. Outcomes were measured using percent of patients screened. A sensitivity analysis was conducted. Findings indicated that the most cost-effective alternative was a targeted reminder. It increased screening by 13% at an incremental cost of $319 per additional patient screened.

Cost-Utility Analysis

A cost-utility analysis (CUA) is a comparative evaluation of two or more interventions in which costs are calculated in dollars and outcomes are calculated in quality of life units. This section focuses on quality of life units (the denominator of the ratio).

A CUA provides information to decision makers not only about the quantity of the outcome (e.g., years of life gained), but also provides information about how individuals perceive the quality of the life years that were gained (Elnitsky & Stone, 2005; Russell, Gold et al., 1996). CUA has been described as a type of CEA in which the health unit considers both quantity and quality (Muennig, 2008; Russell, Gold et al., 1996). There are a number of measures that can be used in a CUA. These include quality adjusted life years (QALYs), disability adjusted life years (DALYs), years of healthy life (YHL), and healthy years equivalent (HYE). The focus of this section is on QALYs because they are the most widely applicable and frequently used measures (Drummond et al., 2005; Russell, Gold et al., 1996).

The QALY was developed as an attempt to measure and value the effect of a change in health status on quality of life. The value of QALYs generally range from 0 (death) to 1 (completely healthy) depending upon the adjustment made for disease or disability (Drummond et al., 2005; Muennig, 2008). There are a number of methodological issues inherent in measuring quality and each issue is open to debate. As an example, who should measure the quality of life after a bilateral mastectomy — a sample of the general community or a sample of individuals who have had or are deciding whether to have a mastectomy? It partly depends upon the nature of the question one is trying to answer. If the issue is the allocation of resources to these interventions versus unrelated health care interventions, perhaps those selected to complete an instrument that measures quality should be drawn from the community because the objective is to obtain a societal preference. However, if the question deals with patients' choices among alternative interventions for breast cancer, measuring the impact of disease on quality of life would best be left to individuals who actually are affected by the disease or condition (Gold et al., 1996; Muennig, 2008; Nord, 1994).

There are a variety of economic methods available to measure a preference for one health state compared to another. In general, the methods were developed to calculate the utility of an outcome based on the probability that the outcome will occur (Drummond et al., 2005; Muennig, 2008). The standard gamble is a frequently used economic method that gauges an individual's preference for the certainty of chronic disease compared to a life and death alternative (Figure 4.1). In the standard gamble, the probability of the life and death alternatives are varied until the respondent is indifferent between the alternatives: (1) the uncertainty of a given probability of death or 1 minus that probability of living in perfect health, as opposed to (2) living in a chronic (but imperfect) health state with certainty.

For example, a patient with mitral valve disease must make a choice. Should the patient have surgery to repair the valve? If otherwise disease free, the surgery might return the patient to perfect health. On the other hand, all surgery has risks and the patient could die during the operation or from surgical complications. Perhaps the patient should elect to do nothing and live within the limitations of the condition? The patient decides that if the chance of dying during surgery is 30% or less, the patient will go ahead with the surgery. If the chance of dying is greater than 30% then the patient will not have surgery but continue in the current health state. At this point, the patient has rated an acceptable quality of life as 70% of perfect health.

In addition to the standard gamble, another commonly used approach is the Time Tradeoff Method, in which participants are offered the choice of varying lengths of life in their current imperfect health state versus a shorter length of life in perfect health. Both the Standard Gamble and the Time Tradeoff Method have produced reliable QALY estimates.

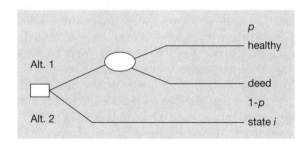

FIGURE 4.1
Standard gamble.
Adapted from *Methods for the economic evaluation of health care programmes*,
M. F. Drummond, M. J. Sculpher, G. W. Torrance, B. J. O'Briend, &
G. L. Stoddart (2005). Oxford University Press, p. 150.

There are also a variety of generic and disease-specific health-related quality of life (HRQL) measures that are currently used (McDowell & Newell, 1996). A discussion of each is beyond the scope of this chapter, but a few examples are: physical disability measurements (e.g., the Medical Outcomes Study Physical Functioning Measure), social health measurements (e.g., the Social Adjustment Scale), and general health status (e.g., the Short Form-36 Health Survey and the Short Form-12 Health Survey). During the last few decades QALYs have gained international acceptance as the outcome of choice in economic CUA studies because they comprise a metric for effect and a preference for that effect (Iglehart, 2010). However, analyses using QALYs are often difficult and expensive.

While QALYs are not a perfect measure, they do represent systematically and objectively collected information from the perspective of affected individuals and societal members that can be used to help decision makers address difficult health care choices. Schickedanz (2010) reported on a symposium sponsored by the Institute of Medicine, the purpose of which was to discuss ways to optimize the value of cancer treatment. There was general agreement that money spent on cancer treatment in the United States far exceeds money spent by other nations, but that the outcomes obtained in this country are not appreciably better than countries spending much less. A survey of oncologists in one New England state revealed that an incremental cost utility of $300,000/QALY would meet their standards for a justifiable intervention. One reason given for this relatively high cost per QALY threshold was that oncologists do not have incentives to choose the less expensive of equally effective treatments, and that their choices do not always consider their patients' quality of life. Members of the symposium agreed that there were steps they could take to improve the value of treatment for their patients. They acknowledged the importance of cost and quality of life in making patient care decisions, and they developed outcome domains, care domains, and patient-centered domains to holistically improve patient health status.

Examples of CUAs are now discussed and are also presented in Table 4.3. Graves et al. (2009) evaluated a 6-month intervention that combined increased nursing and physiotherapy compared to usual care. Potential savings were calculated based on the outcomes determined from an RCT that found patients receiving the intervention had significantly fewer hospital readmissions, emergency room (ER) visits, and significantly increased QALYs. The analysis took a provider perspective and included the cost of nursing assessment and follow up, telephone calls, physical therapy, supplies and material, and the cost of readmission to a hospital or nursing home. The 12-Item Short Form Health Survey (SF-12v2) was used to calculate QALYs. A Markov modeling process, a type of analysis used to make estimations about the state of patients' health at defined periods of time, was used to estimate cost savings at selected endpoints (Muennig, 2008; Petitti, 1994). The authors concluded that the intervention saved $333 (2008 Australian dollars) per patient and increased QALYs by 0.118.

In another example, Handley, Shumway, and Schillinger (2008) determined the cost utility and cost effectiveness of automated telephone self-management support and nursing care compared to usual care in the treatment of patients with type 2 diabetes. This randomized trial was conducted along with an economic analysis and took a health systems perspective. It involved 226 patients from a low-income and ethnically diverse population. Only direct costs were measured and included personnel, supplies and equipment, and overhead. Outcomes were QALYs in the CEA and a 10% increase in meeting disease-specific goals in the CUA. The 12-Item Short Form Health Survey (SF-12) was used to calculate QALYs. Sensitivity analysis was conducted. Findings indicated the program cost $65,167 (U.S. dollars) per QALY when compared to usual care and $558 to increase the percentage of patients meeting exercise goals by 10%. The authors concluded that the program was effective and consistent with other studies of diabetes-related interventions.

Lal et al. (2011) used data from a randomized clinical trial of alternative treatment protocols (stereotactic radiosurgery [SRS] vs. SRS plus whole brain radiation [WBRT]) for patients with brain metastases to conduct both CEAs and CUAs. They developed a decision analysis model and determined the incremental cost per life year saved (LYS) and cost per QALY. Their institutional perspective costs included technical and professional costs. There was a statistically significant difference in the median survival between the two groups. The time trade-off method, using 10-year, 5-year, and 1-year time horizons, was used to determine patient utilities at baseline and at the last time of contact with each patient during the study. Results indicated that compared to SRS plus WBRT, SRS alone had a higher average cost ($74,000 versus $119,000, respectively), but also a higher average effectiveness (0.60 LYS v 1.64 LYS, respectively), with an incremental cost effectiveness ratio (ICER) of $44,231 per LYS, or $41,783 per QALY (using the 10-year horizon). ICER estimates calculated for the 5-year and 1-year time horizons were $43,280/QALY and $44,064/QALY, respectively. Sensitivity analyses indicated robust results, indicating that SRS alone was the more cost-effective treatment arm.

Cost-Benefit Analysis

A cost-benefit analysis (CBA) is a comparative evaluation of two or more interventions in which costs and outcomes are calculated in dollars. The results may be given in a ratio or as dollars saved or lost (Drummond et al., 2005). An advantage of CBAs is that comparisons can be made across disease states and interventions because both costs and outcomes are calculated in dollars. As such, only a CBA asks whether an intervention is worth undertaking. CEAs and CUAs make the implicit assumption that the best of the interventions will be undertaken. Assigning a monetary estimate to morbidity and mortality indicators is technically difficult and it is not something with which many providers in the health care field are comfortable (Garber et al., 1996).

While the number of willingness-to-pay CBA calculations is growing in the health care field, they are far fewer in number than CEAs.

In an example of a CBA, Siddharthan, Nelson, Tiesman, and Chen (2005) combined an observational study along with a CBA to determine the impact of a program designed to reduce the frequency and severity of staff injuries in the Veterans Health Administration (VHA) system (Table 4.3). The 18-month study included 537 nursing personnel and the perspective was the VHA hospital system. Costs included capital costs, training costs, and direct costs associated with treatment of injured nursing personnel and work time lost due to the injuries. The program significantly reduced the annual injury rate from 24 per 100 workers to 16.9 per 100 workers. The program resulted in a $207,000 (U.S. dollars) annualized net benefit stemming from a lower incidence and severity of injuries among nursing personnel. The authors noted that parts of the safety program had been integrated into national occupational health policy.

Economists recommend that, whenever feasible, timing adjustments and sensitivity analyses should be applied to outcomes of care as well as to costs (Drummond et al., 2005). When an economic evaluation is completed, the results of the study along with limitations, implications, and recommendations are submitted in a report to decision makers. Efficiency should not be the only determining factor in deciding among alternative interventions; rather, it is one of many factors in the evaluation process. Other factors include agency policies, legislative mandates, ethical concerns, and input from the general public and support groups (Brosnan & Swint, 2001).

IMPLICATIONS FOR THE APN

Nursing has assumed a limited responsibility in evaluating the efficiency of health care. In a review of nursing literature to determine the quantity and quality of economic evaluations of nursing care, Lämås et al. (2009) found that during a period of 23 years (1984–2007) nurses conducted 115 published studies. Most of the studies (53) related to prevention and treatment with the greatest number (31) focused on wound care. In 78% of the studies the economic method was not discussed, and in 75% the perspective was not provided. The authors attributed the paucity of studies to methodological problems including a lack of nursing outcome indicators.

Economic evaluations are complex and technically difficult. They require specialized knowledge in the disciplines of economics, statistics, epidemiology, and research. Nursing administrators, researchers, and educators have challenged nurses to assume a greater role in appraising the cost effectives of care (Newhouse, 2010; AACN, *DNP Essentials*, 2006; Siegel, 1998; Stone, 1998). The challenge may be addressed in three ways. First, educators must decide how much of an advanced practitioner program should be devoted to disciplines that enable nurses to conduct economic analyses. APNs cannot be all things to all people. As a practical matter, nursing may need to focus on educating the very best practitioners and not on preparing health economists, statisticians, or epidemiologists. Nurses interested in greater participation in economic evaluation may want to take additional courses in economics. Second, nursing programs do need to provide sufficient content to ensure that APNs have a good understanding of fundamental economic concepts and the skill to critique economic evaluations. These abilities will enable APNs to choose the intervention that most effectively and efficiently meets the needs of their patients. Third, APNs bring specialized knowledge to an interdisciplinary team and should collaborate with other health professionals in conducting economic evaluations. A basic grounding in economic concepts and methods will increase the likelihood that APNs will be included in discussions that impact the health status of patients, the health care system, and health policy.

BOX 4.1 INCREMENTAL COST-EFFECTIVENESS OF A REMINDER TELEPHONE CALL

Case Study

The effectiveness of regular eye exams for patients with diabetes mellitus has been established and guidelines developed based on the evidence. In the past, it has been standard to rely on patients to keep track of their own appointments. The APN is a member of an evaluation team that is analyzing the incremental cost-effectiveness of a new program in which patients are contacted by phone to set up an eye exam appointment. To compare the cost and effectiveness of the no program alternative (Method 1) and the reminder telephone call alternative (Method 2) 200 patients were randomly assigned to each group and matched for demographic characteristics and risk factors. Analysis indicated that in Method 1, 55 of 200 patients returned for an appointment, and in Method 2, 120 of 200 patients returned. The cost of contacting patients by phone to set up a screening appointment was $10 per patient with personnel accounting for most of the cost. Determine the cost effectiveness and incremental cost effectiveness of the new program. Would you recommend adopting the new program? Provide a rationale.

Calculations

As there was no cost associated with Method 1, the incremental cost effectiveness of Method 2 versus Method 1 is:

$$\frac{\text{Cost of intervention 2} - \text{Cost of intervention 1}}{\text{Outcome of intervention 2} - \text{Outcome of intervention 1}}$$

or

$$\frac{\$2,000 - 0}{120 - 55} = \frac{\$2,000}{65} = \$30.77 \qquad \text{Per additional patient returned and examined}$$

REFERENCES

Adams, M. E., McCall, N. T., Gray, D. T., Orza, M. J., & Chalmers, T. C. (1992). Economic analysis in randomized control trials. *Medical Care, 30*(3), 231–243.

American Association of Colleges of Nursing. (2006). *The essentials of doctoral education for advanced nursing practice.* Washington, DC: Author.

American Association of Colleges of Nursing. (2011, March 21). *The essentials of master's education in nursing.* Washington, DC: Author.

Ayadi, M. F., Adams, E. K., Melvin, C. L., Rivera, C. C., Gaffney, C. A., Pike, J., ... Ferguson, J. N. (2006). Cost of a smoking cessation counseling intervention for pregnant women: Comparison of three settings. *Public Health Reports, 121,* 120–126.

Brook, R. H., & Lohr, K. N. (1985). Efficacy, effectiveness, variations, and quality. Boundary-crossing research. *Medical Care, 23*(5), 710–722.

Brosnan, C. A., & Swint, J. M. (2001). Cost analysis: Concepts and application. *Public Health Nursing, 18*(1), 13–18.

Brosnan, C. A., Swint, J. M., Upchurch, S. L., Meininger, J. C., Johnson, G., Lee, Y. F., ... Eissa, M. A. (2008). The cost of screening adolescents for overweight and hypertension using a community partnership model. *Public Health Nursing, 25*(3), 235–243.

Buerhaus, P. I. (1998). Milton Weinstein's insights on the development, use, and methodologic problems in cost-effectiveness analysis. *Image: Journal of Nursing Scholarship, 30*(3), 223–228.

Centers for Medicare and Medicaid Services. (2011). Washington, D.C.: U.S. Social Security Administration.

Drummond, M. F., Sculpher, M. J., Torrance, G. W., O'Briend, B. J., & Stoddart, G. L. (2005). *Methods for the economic evaluation of health care programmes.* Oxford: Oxford University Press.

Elnitsky, C. A., & Stone, P. (2005). Patient preferences and cost-utility analysis. *Applied Nursing Research, 18*(2), 74–76.

Finkler, S. A. (1982). The distinction between cost and charges. *Annals of Internal Medicine, 96,* 102–109.

Garber, A. M., Weinstein, M. S., Torrance, G. W., & Kamlet, M. S. (1996). Theoretical foundations of cost-effectiveness analysis. In M. R. Gold, J. E. Siegel, L. B. Russell, & M. C. Weinstein (Eds.), *Cost-effectiveness in health and medicine* (pp. 25–53). New York, NY: Oxford University Press.

Gold, M. R., Patrick, D. L., Torrance, G. W., Fryback, D. G., Hadorn, D. C., Kamlet, M. S., ... Weinstein, M. C. (1996). Identifying and valuing outcomes. In M. R. Gold, J. E. Siegel, L. B. Russell, & M. C. Weinstein (Eds.). *Cost-effectiveness in health and medicine* (pp. 25–53). New York, NY: Oxford University Press.

Graves, N., Courtney, M., Edwards, H., Chang, A., Parker, A., & Finlayson, K. (2009). Cost-effectiveness of an intervention to reduce emergency re-admissions to hospital among older patients. *PLoS ONE, 4*(10), e7455. doi:10.1371/journal.pone.0007455

Handley, M. S., Shumway, M., & Schillinger, D. (2008). Cost-effectiveness of automated telephone self-management support with nurse care management among patients with diabetes. *Annals of Family Medicine, 6*(6), 512–518.

Hardin, G. (1968). The tragedy of the commons. *Science, 162,* 1243–1248.

Herring, A. A., Woolhandler, S., & Himmelstein, D. U. (2008). Insurance Status of U.S. Organ Donors and Transplant recipients: the uninsured give, but rarely receive. *International Journal of Health Services, 38*(4), 641–652.

Hiatt, H. (1975). Protecting the medical commons, who is responsible? *New England Journal of Medicine, 293*(5), 235–241.

Iglehart, J. K. (2010). The political fight over comparative effectiveness research. *Health Affairs, 29*(10), 1757–1760.

Institute of Medicine. (2004). *Care without coverage: Too little, too late.* Washington, DC: National Academics Press. Retrieved from http://www.nap.edu/catalog. php?record_id=10367

Lairson, D. R., DiCarlo, M., Myers, R. E., Wolf, T., Cocroft, J., Sifri, R., ... Wender, R. (2008). Cost-effectiveness of targeted and tailored interventions on colorectal cancer screening use. *Cancer, 112*(4), 779–788.

Lal, L. S., Byfield DaCosta, S., Chang, E., Franzini, L., Miller, L. A., Arbuckle, R., . . . Swint, J. M. (2011). Cost-effectiveness analysis of a randomized study with stereotactic radiosurgery (SRS) versus SRS plus whole brain radiation therapy for patients with brain metastases. *American Journal of Clinical Oncology.* Advance online publication. doi:10.1097/COC.0b013e3182005a8f

Lämås, K., Willman, A., Lindholm, L., & Jacobsson, C. (2009). Economic evaluation of nursing practices: A review of literature. *International Nursing Review, 56*, 13–20.

Lipscomb, J., Weinstein, M. C., & Torrance, G. W. (1996). Time preference. In M. Gold, J. Siegel, L. B. Russell, & M. C. Weinstein (Eds.). *Cost-effectiveness in health and medicine* (pp. 214–246). New York, NY: Oxford University Press.

Luce, R. R., Manning, W. G., Siegel, J. E., & Lipscomb, J. (1996). Estimating costs in cost-effectiveness analysis. In M. Gold, J. Siegel, L. B. Russell, & M. C. Weinstein (Eds.). *Cost-effectiveness in health and medicine* (pp. 176–213). New York, NY: Oxford University Press.

Manning, W. G., Fryback, D. G., & Weinstein, M. C. (1996). Reflecting uncertainty in cost-effectiveness analysis. In M. Gold, J. Siegel, L. B. Russell, & M. C. Weinstein (Eds.). *Cost-effectiveness in health and medicine* (pp. 247–275). New York, NY: Oxford University Press.

McDowell, I., & Newell, C. (1996). *Measuring health.* New York, NY: Oxford University Press.

McIntosh, E., Barlow, J. Davis, H., & Stewart-Brown, S. (2009). Economic evaluation of an intensive home visiting programme for vulnerable families: A cost-effectiveness analysis of a public health intervention. *Journal of Public Health, 31*(3), 423–433.

Muennig, P. (2008). *Cost effectiveness analyses in health: A practical approach.* San Francisco, CA: Jossey-Bass, A Wiley Imprint.

Muennig, P. A., & Glied, S. A. (2010). What changes in survival rates tell us about US health care. *Health Affairs, 29*(11), 1–9. doi:10.1377/hlthall.2010.0073

Newhouse, R. P. (2010). Do we know how much the evidence-based intervention cost? *JONA, 40*(7/8), 296–299.

Nord, E. (1994). The QALY—a measure of social value rather than individual utility? *Economic Evaluation, 3*, 89–93.

Petitti, D. B. (1994). *Meta-analysis, decision analysis and cost-effectiveness analysis.* New York, NY: Oxford University Press.

Porter, M. E. (2010). What is value in health care? *The New England Journal of Medicine, 363*(26), 2477–2481.

Russell, L. B., Gold, M. R., Siegel, J. E., Daniels, N., & Weinstein, M. C. (1996). The role of cost-effectiveness analysis in health and medicine. *JAMA, 276*(14), 1172–1180.

Russell, L. B., Siegel, J. E., Daniels, N., Gold, M. R., Luce, B. R., & Mandelblatt, J. S. (1996). Cost-efffectiveness analysis as a guide to resource allocation in health: roles and limitations. In M. Gold, J. Siegel, L. B. Russell, & M. C. Weinstein (Eds.). *Cost-effectiveness in health and medicine* (pp. 3–24). New York, NY: Oxford University Press.

Schickedanz, A. (2010). Of value: A discussion of cost, communication, and evidence to improve cancer care. *The Oncologist, 15*(Suppl. 1), 73–79.

Siddharthan, K., Nelson, A., Tiesman, H., & Chen, F. (2005, February). Cost effectiveness of a multifaceted program for safe patient handling. *Advances in Patient Safety: From Research to Implementation: (Vol. 3. Implementation Issues).* Rockville, MD: Agency for healthcare Research and Quality.

Siegel, J. E. (1998). Cost-effectiveness analysis and nursing research—is there a fit? *Image: Journal of Nursing Scholarship, 30*(3), 221–222.

Stone, P. W. (1998). Methods for conducting and reporting cost-effectiveness analysis in nursing. *Image: Journal of Nursing Scholarship, 30*(3), 229–234.

Torrance, G. W., Siegel, J. E., & Luce, B. B. (1996). Framing and designing the cost-effectiveness analysis. In M. Gold, J. Siegel, L. B. Russell, & M. C. Weinstein (Eds.). *Cost-effectiveness in health and medicine* (pp. 54–81). New York, NY: Oxford University Press.

Weinstein, M. C., Siegel, J. E., Gold, M. R., Kamlet, M. S., & Russell, L. B. (1996). Recommendations of the panel on cost-effectiveness in health and medicine. *JAMA, 276*(15), 1253–1258.

Weinstein, M. C., & Stason, W. B. (1977). Foundations of cost-effectiveness analysis for health and medical practices. *The New England Journal of Medicine, 296*(13), 716–721.

Williamson, J. W. (1978). *Assessing and improving health care and outcomes: The health accounting approach to quality assurance.* Cambridge, MA: Balinger Publishing Co.

World Bank. (2011). Retrieved from http://search.worldbank.org.

World Health Organization (WHO). Retrieved from http://www.who.int/countries/

FIVE

Evaluating Organizations and Systems

Ann Scanlon-McGinity and Maureen Disbot

> *"Every organization—not just business—needs*
> *one core competency: innovation."*
>
> *Peter Drucker*

INTRODUCTION

For advanced practice nurses (APNs) contemplating career options, the choice of care environments in which to practice is critical. Currently there are limited resources beyond colleagues' recommendations to inform those choices, so it is essential for APNs to have some systematic assessment framework by which to make an informed decision. Selecting an organization or a system in which to practice as an APN requires a systematic review of key indicators that will ensure greater congruency between the organizational and system work environment and that desired by the APN. The complexity of decision making and options requires a thorough investigation of an organization or system prior to interviewing for a position. In this chapter the term "organization" will be used as inclusive of both individual organizations and systems. Using Avedis Donabedian's framework (Glickman, Baggett, Krubert, Peterson, & Schulman, 2007) for assessing a health care organization's performance relative to structure, process, and outcome, the intent of this chapter is to provide a framework for APNs to assess environments in which they potentially might choose to practice. Structure refers to the resources dedicated to provide direct patient care. Such areas as nurse staffing, use of APNs, technologies available to patients, and services provided, as well as special designations provided by external organizations, all reflect the comprehensiveness and quality of care delivered. Achieving Magnet designation from the American Nurse Credentialing Center (ANCC) and accreditation by the Joint Commission (JC) in specialty areas such as stroke and chest pain are examples of an organization's efforts to achieve gold standards in selected areas. Process addresses the organization's reputation for *sustaining* systems of care that are of the highest quality and that are recognized by peers through benchmarking databases. Outcomes data on care effectiveness compare morbidity and mortality with institutions that are similar and who meet threshold targets set by national organizations.

The following areas will be explored to provide the APN with sufficient data for a preliminary decision about the fit with the organization and the value ascribed to the contributions of APNs within that enterprise. The areas addressed include:

- Reputation
- Care outcomes: quality and satisfaction
- Academic and research affiliations
- Professional development
- Compensation and benefits

INVESTIGATING THE ROLE OF THE APNs TO ENSURE SUCCESS

Bryant-Lukosius, Dicenso, Browne, and Pinelli (2004), describe the confusion about the role of the APN as evidenced by misuse of terms, inconsistent titling, misunderstood or undervalued educational preparation, and varied interpretations of its purpose. It is therefore essential that the prospective employer offers full utilization of the APN role of interest (i.e., nurse anesthetist, nurse practitioner, clinical nurse specialist, and nurse midwife), and not merely to serve as a physician replacement or the solution to the reduction in work hours as dictated by the American College of Graduate Medical Education (ACGME) for resident training. There must be an organizational commitment to collaborative and evidence-based practice that includes the development of specific goals for the APN that are measured and shared with both the individual and the organization. Faculty members of the applicant's college, practicing APNs, and the recruiting employer play an integral role in the successful transition of the student APN to the practicing APN. Partnerships with these individuals during the interviewing phase will improve the likelihood of securing compatible employment for both the applicant and the hiring organization.

The following provides an account of one APN's experience in securing a first position as an APN.

> My first interview for a nurse practitioner (NP) position was pretty disappointing. I was scheduled to meet with the Chief Nurse but was only briefly introduced to her and then escorted to a room for a period of four hours where I was interviewed by

a series of administrators, nurse directors, one physician, and the hospital chaplain. The interview questions were all similar and very superficial. There was also some confusion about what my role would be if I were to accept the position. My distinct impression was that this organization had very little understanding of the skills and education of a NP. One of the administrators stated, "We see nurses as one big happy family, they are all cross trained in their units to adjust for patient needs or changes in staffing." I was not entirely discouraged by this interview because it prepared me for the next one. I recognized the importance of making sure I offered future interviewees an opportunity to better understand the scope of practice of the NP and how this role can bring value to their organization.

If you happen to be the first APN to be employed in a facility, be prepared to educate administrators, employees, colleagues, and patients about the scope of practice. This will be most important for other APNs and the collaborating physicians. Frequent communications and collaboration will offer the best opportunities for meeting expectations, achieving your professional goals, and meeting organizational needs. (Personal conversation, July 1, 2011)

Despite the experience described in the interview above, there are many examples of progressive organizations that support the APN as a key member of the clinical team and as an organizational leader. In order to promulgate more widespread understanding and acceptance of the APN role, it is essential to have a common language, described in Table 5.1.

The understanding of "advancement" by prospective employers as the purposeful action taken by the APN to advance patient outcomes through the integration of knowledge and skills can be evaluated simply by asking the interviewers a simple question: "What leadership roles do APNs hold at your

TABLE 5.1
Definitions of Terms Relevant to APN Roles

Term	Definition
Advanced nursing practice or advanced practice	What nurses "do" in the role Involves multiple interacting role domains broadly related to clinical practice, education, research, professional development and organizational leadership (Canadian Association of Nurses in Oncology, 2001) Distinguished from basic practice through specialization, expansion and advancement (American Nurses Association, 1995)
Advanced clinical practice	Clinical care or direct nurse-client interaction (Brown, 1998)

(continued)

TABLE 5.1

Definitions of Terms Relevant to APN Roles (*continued*)

Term	Definition
Advancement	Specialization and expansion of knowledge, skills and role autonomy (American Nurses Association, 1995) Professional activities that lead to innovation and improved nursing care (McGee & Castledine, 2003; Davies & Hughes, 1995) Commitment to a nursing orientation to practice Synthesis Integration of practical, theoretical and research knowledge (American Nurses Association, 1995) Purposeful integration and application of role competencies related to clinical practice, education, research, leadership and professional development to improve patient health (Davies & Hughes, 1995; Hamric, 2000)
Advanced practice nursing	The whole field of a specific type of nursing, namely advanced nursing practice (Brown, 1998; Royal College of Nursing Australia, 2000; Styles & Lewis, 2000) Includes APN roles, APN environments and environmental factors affecting role development, implementation and evaluation
Advanced practice nursing roles	A variety of roles in which nurses function at an advanced level of practice Roles that include all domains of advanced nursing practice Require graduate education, practice experience, licensure and certification
Advanced practice nursing environments and environmental factors	Local conditions: organizational structures and culture of the work environment Society: values, expectations, demands and needs for health care Health care system: workforce, practice trends and economy Government: funding health care policies, legislation Nursing profession: knowledge production, education, practice, regulatory and credentialing mechanisms and political activities Advanced practice nursing community: advanced practice nurses, educational institutions, specialty organizations and social networks (Brown, 1998; Hamric, 2000; Read, 1999; Roy & Martinez, 1983; Styles & Lewis, 2000)

Bryant-Lukosiu et al. (2004).

organization?" or "How does a new APN move from novice to expert in this organization?" If your prospective employer does not have a well thought out and credible answer to these two questions, the organization might not be a good fit if the APN has aspirations for advancement and professional development. The environmental conditions, which include structure, culture, professional development, and reimbursement models for APNs, offer another focus for the APN's evaluation of compatible organizations and their successful implementation of the APN role, as well as the perceived "value" provided by the APN as a member of the healthcare team. To access detailed information on organizational structure, one can review the American Hospital Association (AHA) surveys (http://www.ahasurvey.org/taker/asindex). This self-report survey was completed by 4851 hospitals in 2010 and includes detailed financials, bed size, and services offered. It also provides staffing and physician data in great detail as part of the overall organizational structure. The AHA survey is used extensively for research and benchmarking purposes. It offers a comprehensive, objective review for anyone interested in this type of evaluation.

Bryant-Lukosius et al. (2004) provide the detailed definitions for the APN to utilize, but it is ultimately the APN seeking employment who will determine her or his own career path. In the book *Outliers*, Malcolm Gladwell offers numerous examples of highly successful individuals who exceed traditional performance not because of their education, ambition, or hard work but through the *interconnection* of the individual, the community in which they work, and the environment that supports the work. The most well-suited organization will be the ones that provide the best connection between personal ability and meaningful work (Gladwell, 2000).

Szanton, Mihaly, Alhusen, and Becker (2010) provide a structured evaluation tool utilizing categories for patient, colleague, and clinic assessments for the new APN graduate.

Table 5.2 provides an organized series of questions for the APN's consideration during the interviewing and the decision-making process.

TABLE 5.2

Patient, Colleague, and Clinical Factors: Questions to Ask When Interviewing

Patient Factors	Colleague Factors	Clinical Factors
• What type of practice setting is most enjoyable to you?	• What considerations are provided for mentorship?	• What are the productivity expectations and what considerations are given to novice APNs?
• What patient population are you seeking to care for?	• Does the practice style of providers foster a learning environment?	• Does the mission of the practice setting support your goals and values?

(*continued*)

TABLE 5.2
Patient, Colleague, and Clinical Factors: Questions to Ask When Interviewing
(*continued*)

Patient Factors	Colleague Factors	Clinical Factors
• What is the typical acuity level of patients served?	• What is the composition of providers?	• Is the model of delivery of care conducive to your practice style?
• How does the level of resources impact your ability to provide care?	• What types of clinical support staff are available for patient care?	• What type of technology is available, and how will that support your learning needs?
	• Does the setting have experience utilizing APNs for provision of care?	• Are there on-call requirements, and what support mechanisms are in place?
		• Will supervision of ancillary staff be an expectation?
		• Is the practice setting one that supports preceptor opportunities of health care providers?

Swanton, S,L., et al. (2010). Taking charge of the challenge. Factors to consider when taking your first nurse practitioner job. *Journal of the American Academy of Nurse Practitioners*, *22*, (2010) 356–360 © 2010. American Academy of Nurse Practitioners.

Consideration of each of these three domains (e.g., patient, colleague, and clinical) provides additional structure to the evaluation process. The evaluation should be supplemented by the feedback received from experienced APNs on staff and other staff and physicians who may be employed within the organization of interest.

REPUTATION

A variety of external reference groups provide summary data related to excellence in clinical performance, which can serve as a benchmark against which all health care organizations can critique their performances. Listed below are examples of reputational entities that prospective APNs might critique when assessing the reputation of a particular organization.

U.S. News and World Report Rankings

In 1990, *U.S. News and World Report* introduced "Best Hospitals" as a resource for families seeking help with medical concerns to help them select those hospitals that might provide the best level of care for their specific medical issues (www.rti.org/besthospitals). The annual report ranks hospitals in 16 specialties and is available to anyone wishing to purchase the publication at any newsstand or book store. Hospital rankings are primarily based on quality data as well as physician survey information. Factored into hospital rankings are such metrics as nurse staffing, use of technologies, and external recognition by organizations such as the American Nurse Credentialing Center (ANCC). These hospital rankings serve the APN in assessing specialty practice as well as reputation scores (http://health.usnews.com/best-hospitals/rankings).

Magnet Designation

Of the 17 hospitals identified in *U.S. News and World Report* "Best Hospitals" in 2011, 14 were Magnet-designated hospitals. Magnet criteria identify five domains and over 60 sources of evidence that are essential for creating an environment in which nurses thrive and innovate. Leading these domains is transformational leadership, which addresses the quality of nursing leadership in an organization. A nurse leader (i.e., Chief Nurse Executive) is one who effectively communicates vision and the role of the nurse in transforming health care processes, and establishes a strategy plan that speaks to the future direction of nursing efforts as hallmarks of a well-led nursing organization. Outcomes of this leadership will be sensitive to the effective positioning of APNs within the nursing structure in ways that can influence program innovation and quality outcomes for patients and families (http://www.nursecredentialing.org/Magnet.aspx).

Magnet designation and The Pathway to Excellence Program offered by the ANCC are indicators of a nursing enterprise that is focused on nurses, quality, service, and innovation in care. The initial designation is preceded by what has been referred to as the "Magnet journey," which is when an organization engages in a rigorous self-assessment to determine if it meets Magnet criteria. The self-assessment is followed by corrective action in areas that need improvement with the goal of establishing and sustaining a Magnet culture. Once an organization believes it is ready to apply, an extensive written report based on the forces of magnetism and evidence are submitted for review. A site visit is scheduled after review of the written documentation. For successful organizations, Magnet designation is awarded for a period of 4 years; annual reports are submitted to demonstrate the sustainability of the Magnet culture and high-quality outcomes.

A rigorous documentation system that tracks performance on nurse-sensitive indicators with corrective action plans must be demonstrated for a 4-year period prior to every re-designation. This is followed by an onsite visit by a team of trained appraisers who spend several days with nursing staff and APNs in their areas of specialty, critiquing their work outputs and the environments in which care is provided. The rigors of this process account for the fact that only about 4% of the nation's hospitals achieve Magnet designation. Effective Magnet-designated organizations have 3 to 5 year nursing strategic plans that address the following elements: collaborative patient care delivery; workplace environment; community presence; evidence-based practice and research; innovation and technology; and financial stewardship (http://www.methodisthealth.com/basic.cfm?id=36818).

Fortune 100 Best Companies to Work For

On an annual basis, the Great Places to Work Institute publishes the list of the Top 100 Best Companies to Work For nationally in *Fortune* magazine. In addition to businesses, this list contains hospital organizations that, via random employee survey, have indicated their work environment is one that reflects a partnership between employer and employee and provides employees with unique and innovative programming reflective of common values. A website (http://money.cnn.com/magazines/fortune/bestcompanies/2011/full_list/) provides a comprehensive review of these organizations and serves the APN well to determine if the hospital/organization in which the individual is considering employment is listed. The number of hospitals achieving this distinction is very limited.

CARE OUTCOMES: EXTERNAL COMPARISONS ON QUALITY AND PATIENT SATISFACTION

In the current age of transparency, there is no shortage of data for an objective review of an organization's performance. Many of the outcomes and process measures collected in health care organizations are abstracted from administrative databases used by payers; some of these data are published routinely. There are far more options for inpatient comparisons, although data on the outpatient environment are improving. Many states like Maryland, Pennsylvania, California, Minnesota, and Virginia have extensive data and report significant outcomes. Payers, including Center for Medicare and Medicaid (CMS), Managed Care, and Fee for Service, have additional reporting capabilities that are often utilized by employers to make choices for their employee health care needs. The Hospital Compare website (http://www.hospitalcompare.hhs.gov/) provides the data for public review. Some of the datasets available include the following.

Core Measures

In early 1999, the Joint Commission (JC) solicited input from a wide variety of stakeholders (e.g., clinical professionals, health care provider organizations, state hospital associations, health care consumers) and convened a Cardiovascular Conditions Clinical Advisory Panel, which was charged to address the potential focus areas for core measures for hospitals. In May 2001, the JC announced four initial core measurement for hospitals, which included acute myocardial infarction (AMI) and heart failure (HF). Simultaneously, The JC worked with the CMS on the AMI and HF sets that were common to both organizations. The CMS and the JC worked to align the measure specifications for use in the 7th Scope of Work and for JC-accredited hospitals. Hospitals began collecting AMI measures for patient discharges beginning July 1, 2002.

In November of 2003, the CMS and the JC began to work to precisely and completely align these common measures; they are now identical. This resulted in the creation of one common set of measure specification documentations known as the Specifications Manual for National Hospital Inpatient Quality Measures to be used by both organizations. The Manual contains a common (i.e., identical) data dictionary, measurement information forms, algorithms, and other items. The goal is to minimize data collection efforts for these common measures and focus efforts on the use of data to improve the health care delivery processes.

The Core Measures sets include:

- Acute Myocardial Infarction (AMI)
- Children's Asthma Care (CAC)
- Heart Failure (HF)
- Hospital-Based Inpatient Psychiatric Services (HBIPS)
- Hospital Outpatient Department Measures
- Perinatal Care (PC)
- Pneumonia (PN)
- Stroke (STK)
- Surgical Care Improvement Project (SCIP)

The core measures are based on the currently approved evidence-based guidelines adopted by the JC, the National Quality Forum (NQF), and the CMS.

The success of core measures requires a multi-modal approach with a major focus on a collaborative practice model, the nursing process, and excellent technological support. An APN can evaluate a potential employer's effectiveness by visiting the hospital website and by comparing it to other organizations for performance in any or all of these measures. The APN should bring this information to the interview to discuss with the interviewer, as well as to discuss the important role that the APN will have in the successful achievement of these measures. A complete list of inpatient and outpatient measures with definitions can be found on the Hospital Quality Alliance website (http://www.hospitalqualityalliance.org/hospitalqualityalliance/qualitymeasures/qualitymeasures.html).

Hospital Acquired Conditions (HACs)

These are serious conditions that patients may acquire during an inpatient hospital stay. If hospitals follow proper procedures and use evidence-based guidelines to treat and care for patients, patients are less likely to acquire these conditions. The APN may wish to collect information for several organizations to determine if the potential employer has a disproportionate share of poor outcomes. Organizations who are outliers may have different processes from best practices or significant process failures. If the APN is prepared to review this information during the interview, be sure to include some positive results along with negative findings for balance. This offers a good opportunity to determine the organization's approach to evidence-based practice and effective deployment of those practices.

Health Care-Associated Infections (HAIs)

HAIs are infections caused by a wide variety of both common and unusual bacteria, fungi, and viruses during the course of receiving medical care. Medical advances have brought lifesaving care to patients, yet many of those advances come with a risk of HAIs. These infections can be devastating and even deadly. Currently, the infections that are being reported publically are blood stream infections (BSI), urinary tract infections (UTI), and ventilator-associated pneumonias (VAP). All of these infections carry significant morbidity and mortality; therefore the APN should be aware of any federal or state data available in the area of interest to assess expected quality of care.

Private Organizations

There are also many other private organizations such as Health Grade (http://www.healthgrades.com/business/services/) and Thompson Reuter (http://www.100tophospitals.com/top-national-hospitals/) who have developed proprietary methodologies to analyze public datasets to evaluate the quality of health care providers. Review the internet sites of all potential employers. This is where the APN will be able to gather the most recently published information related to clinical quality outcomes for that employer. Insight will also be gained about the organizational culture if the internet sites are populated with current outcomes.

According to The Commonwealth Fund (Collins & Davis, 2006), transparency and better public information on cost and quality are essential for three reasons: 1) to help providers improve by benchmarking their performance against others; 2) to encourage private insurers and public programs to reward quality and efficiency; and 3) to help patients make informed choices about their care. Transparency is also important to level the playing field through disclosure of accurate and comparable information on how all components of patient care are addressed. For example, the widespread practice of charging patients different prices for the same care is inherently inequitable, especially when the uninsured are charged more than other patients. Accurate information is critical for the expected level of transparency related to health care.

Hospital Consumer Assessment of Healthcare Providers and System (HCAHPS)

The Hospital Consumer Assessment of Healthcare Providers and System (HCAHPS) survey is the first national, standardized, publicly reported survey of patients' perspectives of hospital care. HCAHPS, also known as the CAHPS® Hospital Survey, is a survey instrument and data collection methodology for *measuring patients' perceptions of their hospital experience*. While many hospitals have collected information on patient satisfaction for their own internal use, until HCAHPS, there was no national standard for collecting and publicly reporting information about patients' experience of care that allowed valid comparisons to be made across hospitals locally, regionally. and nationally (http://www.cms.gov/HospitalQualityInits/30_HospitalHCAHPS.asp).

Table 5.3 provides a brief description and website information for publically reported data that can be reviewed in advance of screening potential employers and in preparation for scheduled interviews.

TABLE 5.3

Website for Publically Reported Data About Hospital Performance

Health Care Acquired Conditions	Source System
Foreign substance accidentally left inside patient during a procedure	http://www.hospitalcompare.hhs.gov/
Falls (codes are not actually for "falls" but for potential adverse events or injuries occurring as the result of falls; injuries that should not occur during a patient's hospitalization). The generic categories of coded injuries include: fractures, dislocations, intracranial injury, crushing injury, burns, and other and unspecified effects of external causes	http://www.hospitalcompare.hhs.gov/
Air embolism	http://www.hospitalcompare.hhs.gov/
Blood incompatibility	http://www.hospitalcompare.hhs.gov/

(continued)

TABLE 5.3
Website for Publically Reported Data About Hospital Performance (*continued*)

Health Care Acquired Conditions	Source System
Venous thromboembolism (VTE) after hip and knee replacement. Although VTE includes deep vein thrombosis (DVT) and pulmonary embolism (PE), CMS has only selected PE codes to which this payment policy applies at this time	http://www.hospitalcompare. hhs.gov/
Poor glycemic control; i.e., ketoacidosis and coma (hypoglycemic and hypo-osmolar).	http://www.hospitalcompare. hhs.gov/
Health Care-Associated Infections	Source System
CR-BSI (vascular catheter-associated infection)	http://www.hospitalcompare. hhs.gov/
CA-UTI	http://www.hospitalcompare. hhs.gov/
VAP	http://www.hospitalcompare. hhs.gov/
SSI: Specific orthopedic infections	http://www.hospitalcompare. hhs.gov/
SSI: CABG medialstinitis	http://www.hospitalcompare. hhs.gov/
SSI: Bariatric surgery for morbid obesity; laparoscopic gastric bypass and gastroenterostomy	Internal source file: Enterprise Datamart, via CMS criteria
HCAHPS (Patient-Mix Adjustments)	Source System
Communication with nurses	http://www.cms.gov/ HospitalQualityInits/30_ HospitalHCAHPS.asp
Communication with doctors	http://www.cms.gov/ HospitalQualityInits/30_ HospitalHCAHPS.asp
Responsiveness of hospital staff	http://www.cms.gov/ HospitalQualityInits/30_ HospitalHCAHPS.asp
Pain management	http://www.cms.gov/ HospitalQualityInits/30_ HospitalHCAHPS.asp
Communication about medicines	http://www.cms.gov/ HospitalQualityInits/30_ HospitalHCAHPS.asp

(*continued*)

TABLE 5.3

Website for Publically Reported Data About Hospital Performance (*continued*)

Health Care Acquired Conditions	Source System
Cleanliness of hospital environment	http://www.cms.gov/ HospitalQualityInits/30_ HospitalHCAHPS.asp
Quietness of hospital environment	http://www.cms.gov/ HospitalQualityInits/30_ HospitalHCAHPS.asp
Recommend to friends and family	http://www.cms.gov/ HospitalQualityInits/30_ HospitalHCAHPS.asp
From internally developed documents at TMH.	

Advance knowledge of these hospital quality measures will provide an excellent platform for discussion about the impact that the APN can make to organizational performance and financial reimbursement. Such a discussion can help the APN in the selection process for potential employers.

Similarly, the Physician Quality Reporting Initiative (PQRI) offers additional opportunity for physicians and other eligible practitioners like NPs, nurse midwives, nurse anesthetists, and clinical nurse specialists to participate in a claims-based reporting system of specific quality measures for which additional reimbursement will be awarded to each practitioner who reaches a high level of achievement (a list of eligible participants is provided in the CMS document http://www.cms.gov/PQRS/).The 2009 PQRI experience report presented in Table 5.4 can be reviewed by specialty and other type of providers. The MD/DO participation exceeded all other providers as did their incentive payments.

TABLE 5.4

Physician Quality Reporting System Incentive by Specialty for All Reporting Methods

Specialty	# TIN/NPI	Minimum	Maximum	Mean	Median	Total	% Total National Incentive
Total	119,804	$0.08	$132,213	$1,955	$939	$234,282,572	100.00%
MD/DO	92,189	$0.08	$132,213	$2,274	$1,236	$209,676,569	89.50%

SUMMARY

This chapter has taken a different approach to evaluation of organizations and systems in that it has considered evaluation from the perspective of an APN interested in securing a position within an organization or system friendly to APN practice. Through a review of the APN role, the various facets of the APN role were examined to better understand the significant and unique contributions that an APN can make to an organization. It is important that the APN find the right match when seeking a position in practice so that desired career opportunities and professional development are available. To assist the APN, an evaluation framework was provided that included the following characteristics of an organization/system: reputation; care outcomes such as quality and satisfaction; academic and research affiliations; professional development; and compensation and benefits. By applying this framework, the APN can better evaluate opportunities that best meet her or his professional and career aspirations.

REFERENCES

American Nurses Association. (1995). *Nursing's social policy statement*. Silver Spring, MD: Author.

Brown, S. (1998). A framework for advanced practice nursing. *Journal of Professional Nursing, 14*, 157–164.

Bryant-Lukosiu, S. D., Dicenso, A., Browne, G., & Pinelli, J. (2004). Advanced practice nursing roles: Development, implementation, and evaluation. *Journal of Advanced Nursing, 48*, 519–529.

Canadian Association of Nurses in Oncology. (2001). *Standards of care, roles in oncology nursing, role competencies*. Kanata, Ontario, Canada: Author.

Collins, S. R., & Davis, K. (2006). Transparency in health care: The time has come. *The Commonwealth Fund*. Retrieved from http://www.commonwealthfund.org/Content/Publications/Testimonies/2006/Mar/Transparency-in-Health-Care—The-Time-Has-Come.aspx

Davies, B., & Hughes, A. M. (1995). Clarification of advanced nursing practice: Characteristics and competencies. *Clinical Nurse Specialist, 9*, 156–160.

Gladwell, M. (2000). *The tipping point: How little things can make a big difference*. Boston, MA: Little, Brown.

Glickman, S. W., Baggett, K. A., Krubert, C. G., Peterson, E. D., & Schulman, K. A. (2007). Promoting quality: The health-care organization from a management perspective. *International Journal for Quality in Health-Care, 19*(6), 341–348.

McGee, P., & Castledine, G. (2003). *Advanced nursing practice* (2nd ed). Oxford, UK: Blackwell.

Read, S. M. (1999). Nurse-led care: The importance of management support. *Nursing Research, 5*, 408–421.

Roy, C., & Martinez, C. (1983). A conceptual framework for CNS practice. In A. B. Hamric & J. A. Spross (Eds.), *The clinical nurse specialist in theory and practice* (pp. 3–20) New York, NY: Gruen & Stratton.

Royal College of Nursing Australia (2000). *Advanced practice nursing*. Retrieved from http:// www.rcan.org.au/content/advancedpracticenursing.gtml

Styles, M., & Lewis, C. (2000). Conceptualizations of advanced nursing practice. In A. B. Hamric, J. A. Spross, & C. M. Hanson (Eds.). *Advanced nursing practice: An integrative approach* (pp. 33–51). Philadelphia, PA: W.B. Saunders.

Szanton, S. L., Mihaly, L. K., Alhusen, J., & Becker, K. L. (2010). Taking charge of the challenge: Factors to consider in taking your first nurse practitioner job. *Journal of the American Academy of Nurse Practitioners, 22*(7), 356–360.

SIX

Evaluating Health Care Information Systems and Patient Care Technology

Sharon McLane

*"The problems that exist in the world today cannot be solved by
the same level of thinking that created them."*

Albert Einstein

INTRODUCTION

This chapter discusses the role of the APN in the assessment of various types
of technologies and information systems used by health care providers and
patients. The purpose of this chapter is to equip the APN with increased
knowledge of: (1) tenets of information technology evaluation; and (2) effective partnerships and collaborations with informaticians and other members
of the information systems team.

The first section addresses the framework of informatics and
informaticians within the context of the clinical environment. It includes the
following topics:

- BL Informatics and the role of the advanced practice informatician
- The collaborative relationship of the APN and informaticians
- The national mandate for electronic health records (EHR) and implications
  of reimbursement for eligible hospitals and providers
- The scope of the term "information technology" (IT)

The second part of the chapter discusses the specific areas in which APNs can make effective contributions in the evaluation of health care and information technologies including:

▪ Informatics competency as a basic tenet of effective use and evaluation of information technology and information systems
▪ Electronic personal health record (ePHR) and recommended evaluation criteria
▪ Recommended guidelines to support patients' searches for authentic health care information on the Internet
▪ Ergonomic evaluation of the work environment with respect to computer technology
▪ Evaluation of computerized patient care equipment

INFORMATICS AND ADVANCED PRACTICE INFORMATICIANS

Adding informatics to the discussion of evaluation appends an interesting and important domain of consideration. The discussion begins by defining informatics, specifically nursing informatics, and the relationship between APNs and informatics practitioners. The American Nurses Association (ANA) defines nursing informatics (NI) as "a specialty that integrates nursing science, computer science, and information science to manage and communicate data, information, knowledge, and wisdom in nursing practice," with the goal of improving the "health of populations, communities, families, individuals by optimizing information management and communication" (American Nurses Association [ANA], 2008, p. 1). The key concept of the ANA definition is the *management and communication of data, information, knowledge, and wisdom to improve health.* Informatics embraces IT in its multiple facets as a *tool* that is purposed to enhance information management and knowledge discovery. Much of the practice of informatics is devoted to the design of an information system. Advanced practice informaticians are also involved in informatics research and the discovery of knowledge and understanding to serve as models that are more effective, seamless, and transparent in the delivery of quality patient care and improved patient outcomes.

Preparation for informatics practice has not been standardized to date. Nurses may begin informatics practice through on-the-job training, completion of an informatics certificate program, and/or completion of a degree-granting program at the bachelor's, master's, or doctoral degree level. Degree domains include health informatics, health care informatics, clinical informatics, nursing informatics, and similar informatics domains (American Medical Informatics Association [AMIA], 2011). The common thread among these entry-to-practice levels is the creation of tools that practitioners can use to promote patient safety, enhance the quality of care delivery, promote health maintenance and disease prevention, and improve outcomes for individuals and populations.

Frequently, the role of the informatician focuses on clinical information system configuration and building in preparation for system implementation. Informaticians who have completed an undergraduate or graduate program are prepared to embrace other important dimensions that are fundamental to developing an information system that effectively supports critical thinking and decision making. These dimensions include:

- Assessment of the socio-technical (e.g., the convergence of people, relationships, systems, and organizational culture) facets of an IT implementation, and the transformations that are deeply embedded in its implementation
- Assessment and management of the human-computer interface; that is, creating positive, intuitive, error "free" experiences for practitioners as they use the technology
- Assessment of current workflow, identifying opportunities for streamlining processes and for development of new workflows in the context of the IT system
- Application of informatics science to domains such as the alignment of cognitive needs of practitioners and the implications of these needs to application design
- Strategic planning that anticipates and positions the organization for the cultural and practice transformation that is associated with the implementation of IT and information systems
- System design that is aligned with the information management and knowledge management needs and characteristics of the organization. (American Medical Informatics Association [AMIA] Nursing Informatics Work Group, 2009; Greenes & Shortliffe, 2009; Gruber, Cummings, Leblanc, & Smith, 2009; Health Information Management Systems Society [HIMSS] Nursing Informatics, 2011; Koppel, Wetterneck, Telles, & Karsh, 2008; McLane & Turley, 2011).

National Mandate for Electronic Health Records (EHRs)

We are living in the digital information age. Health care adopted IT to support the financial imperatives of the organization in the 1970s. However, the complexities of patient care, the multiple environments in which health care is delivered, the diverse patient populations, and the variability of resources of the health care industry resulted in a much more tentative approach to embracing IT for documentation, display, and storage of clinical data. A few early adopters began the journey to digital clinical information systems in the late 1960s, and the number of hospitals and health care systems using IT for clinical documentation slowly increased over the next 4 decades. As recently as 2008, the number of physician office practices with electronic patient records was estimated to be between 17% and 25%. By 2009, less than 8% of U.S. hospitals had implemented computerized provider order entry (CPOE) and less than 4% of hospitals had "closed-loop medication administration"; that is, the seamless alignment of CPOE, pharmacy review, eMAR (electronic medication administration record), and positive patient identification with bar code or radio frequency technology (PPID; HIMSS Analytics, 2010).

National health care policy, as established in the American Recovery and Reinvestment Act (ARRA) of 2009, provided direction to the Centers for Medicare and Medicaid Services (CMS) to responsively create meaningful use rules and criteria for eligible providers and eligible hospitals. CMS also issued criteria for certification of EHRs, and eligible providers and eligible hospitals must report meaningful use of data from a certified EHR by 2015 (Obama, 2009). Beginning in 2015, Medicare payments to eligible providers and eligible hospitals that do not demonstrate meaningful use will be reduced, and the level of reimbursement will continue to decline in subsequent years (CMS, 2011). Recognizing the significant cost associated with implementation of EHRs, CMS offered incentive payments to eligible providers and eligible hospitals, beginning in 2011 and running through 2015. Eligible providers and eligible hospitals that do not successfully demonstrate meaningful use by 2015 would experience payment adjustments to their Medicare reimbursement. These reimbursement changes have created a compelling inducement to reluctant or uncertain health care organizations and eligible providers to embrace IT, specifically the EHR. Since mid-2010, eligible providers and eligible hospitals have accelerated plans for implementation of an EHR, with an initial focus on achieving meaningful use.

Collaboration between APNs and nurse informaticians creates an ideal partnership for the effective use of and design of a clinical information system. The nursing knowledge, clinical expertise, and experience of APNs, in combination with the nursing knowledge, informatics knowledge, and experience of informaticians, merge together to inform the design of a database that collects the information necessary to provide excellent patient care. The synergy of clinical subject matter experts and informatics subject matter experts establishes a harmony of design and function. The APN's expert clinical knowledge and understanding of the data necessary to support clinical assessment, critical thinking, ongoing modification of the plan of care, and patient education are essential to the design of an effective health care information system that will be useful to and usable by practitioners. The nurse informatician carefully evaluates the knowledge and information needs defined by the APN in the context of factors such as future workflow, data visualization, cognition, system navigation, training, practitioner adoption of the system, and data reporting needs.

An interesting and important dimension of the design of an EHR information system is the duality of purpose. The primary focus of an EHR is the individual patient and the information that is necessary to provide effective and efficacious care for that individual. The second, yet still very powerful purpose of an EHR system, is related to the data stored by the system, which can be used to evaluate practice, quality of care, outcomes, and many other dimensions for patient populations. Careful design of the system and thoughtful, intentional data input will create a database that can inform evidence-based practice and provide highly powered data regarding quality of care and patient outcomes. While the quality of care for the individual who has presented for care is the primary focus of the moment, a system that is thoughtfully designed to support data input and data visualization by practitioners who understand and respect the importance and value of the prescribed data input workflow has the potential to create a robust evidence-based database.

IT as a Communication Tool

IT refers to the tools – software, hardware, and communication devices – that support the communication and management of data and information. Computers and computer software are central to IT, and it is important to recognize that the presence of the computer and the software may not be immediately apparent to the user. IT extends beyond the traditional computer to include: smart IV pumps; cellular and analog telephones; text messaging; email; social networking systems such as Facebook, Twitter, and YouTube; point of care testing and data collection devices; patient education databases; online procedure manuals; scheduling and productivity management systems; and voice communication systems such as smart phones and mobile wireless communication systems.

Pen and paper, which are familiar to all, are also a form of IT, as are the signal flags used by naval ships, and Morse code. Each of these examples is a form of communication, and it is important to ensure that the communication of information is the focus of attention, rather than the tools used to spread that information. By reframing the concept of IT as tools used for the purpose of communication of data and information, new horizons are disclosed. The perception of IT as a *tool* rather than as a goal is important. IT projects require a significant focus on the technology development and implementation process. However, the purpose of the tool must be the outcome of the project or we have failed our practitioner customers.

INFORMATICS COMPETENCY

The health care agenda of the United States virtually ensures that clinical information will be digitally recorded and stored (Office of the National Coordinator for Health Information Technology [ONC], 2011). CMS's meaningful use rules signal possible new characterizations and understanding of evidence-based practice. The dominance of digital information has been characterized as an information tsunami (Vastag, 2011). Research has established that as recently as 2007, nearly 94% of available information is digitally stored (Hilbert & Lopez, 2011). These concepts and facts illustrate that the development and maintenance of basic computer skills is no longer a choice and has become a basic life skill, similar to the use of an ATM or paying for groceries with the use of a debit card.

The digitization of information demands that health care practitioners develop the ability to recognize the need for information, locate the information, and effectively evaluate, manipulate, and use the information; and it requires computer literacy and information literacy skills (Association of College and Research Libraries, 2000). Computer literacy and information literacy skills are generally referred to as informatics competencies. Informatics competencies are new or significantly revised skills for care providers who were born prior to 1980. Those earlier generations are often referred to as digital immigrants in comparison to those born after 1980, who are characterized as digital natives (Prensky, 2001).

Integration of informatics competencies into nursing education has been recommended since the mid-1990s (Staggers, Gassert, & Curran, 2001); however, implementation and adoption of these recommendations has occurred more slowly than anticipated. The growing importance of informatics competency served as the catalyst for an invitational summit of nursing leaders in practice, education, informatics, technology, information system vendors, government, and other key stakeholder entities from across the United States in the fall of 2006. The focus of the summit was the development of a vision for the nursing profession that embraces IT to improve practice, patient safety, and patient outcomes. The outcomes of the summit are included the Technology Informatics Guiding Education Reform (TIGER) report. As the work of the summit evolved, a 10-year vision and a 3-year action plan were developed (TIGER, 2007, 2009). In 2007, nine action items were defined and subsequently assigned to one of nine collaboratives. The development of computer literacy skills and information literacy skills by nurses is the focus of one of these nine collaboratives. The outcome of informatics competency is the preparation of nurses to understand and competently use the EHR to improve the health care of each patient and, ultimately, the health care of our nation. A brief summary of the collaboratives and their purpose is presented in Table 6.1.

APNs are in an excellent position to observe the informatics competency skills of the nurses with whom they work. TIGER recommends that all practicing nurses demonstrate basic informatics skills, such as the ability to:

■ Access, send, and add attachments to email
■ Use the Microsoft Windows operation system, such as starting applications, opening files, saving files, use of the taskbar and desktop, etc.
■ Prepare, modify, and print a document in a word processing software application

TABLE 6.1

TIGER Collaboratives

Collaborative	Purpose
Standards and Interoperability	Improve patient care by promoting standardized nursing data, which will enable data mining and will facilitate measurement and comparison of nursing interventions and patient outcomes. Interoperability will assist in communication and data sharing between disparate information systems.
National Health IT Agenda	Increase nursing visibility and participation in the development of national health care policies.
Informatics Competencies	Identify the skills necessary for nurses to effectively use an EHR, to use and contribute to evidence-based practice, and to efficiently access and use information. Recommended competencies include basic computer competency, information literacy, and information management.
Education and Faculty Development	Embed informatics competencies, theories, and research throughout the nursing curriculum and at all educational levels. Encourage funding of informatics curriculum development by foundations. Increase the informatics competency of faculty.
Staff Development	Promote development of cost-effective resources and programs that foster IT innovation, and that promote development of the informatics competency of the practicing nurse.
Leadership Development	Heighten awareness and understanding of nurse leaders regarding the value of information technology and the importance of developing their personal informatics competency to lead the drive for improved patient safety, care delivery, and patient outcomes.
Usability and Clinical Application Design	Promote user-focused system design and adoption of proven system integration, usability, and application design principles in the development of clinical information systems.
Virtual Demonstration Center	Two virtual conferences were held to increase visibility of the actual and potential benefits to be realized from IT, which will: enhance practice and improve patient care; demonstrate best practices; and improve quality and safety. Future goals include development of a virtual environment, such as Second Life®, for education about the features and benefits of information technology (Linden Resarch Inc., 2011).

(continued)

TABLE 6.1
TIGER Collaboratives (*continued*)

Collaborative	Purpose
Consumer Empowerment and Personal Health Records	Empower patients to increase understanding of their health, to effectively prevent disease, and to manage their chronic diseases. Nurses need to understand ePHR tools so that they can knowledgeably discuss the ePHR options and benefits with the patient and their family or care giver.

Adapted from *Collaborating to Integrate Evidence and Informatics into Nursing Practice and Education: An Executive Summary* by TIGER (2009).

- Copy and paste functions in various applications
- Ability to prepare a simple spreadsheet and use simple formulas, filter data, manipulate data, and prepare a simple graph or chart

When informatics skills are inadequate or missing, APNs may wish to champion informatics skill acquisition, thus positioning the staff for future success. Often there are computer and information management continuing education program options available within the community at local high schools, vocational schools, colleges, or universities. A wide variety of distance education program are available online, which can generally to be completed at the learner's pace. The TIGER Initiative suggested several options for the development of informatics competency, including the European Computer Driving License (ECDL) Foundation, the HIMSS, and the American Library Association (TIGER, 2009, p. 16).

ePHR for Patients

Electronic personal health records (ePHR) are a more recent entry in the electronic health record field and, relatively speaking, have received much less attention than the development and installation of EHR systems. A generally accepted definition of ePHR and agreement regarding standards for the content, functionality, and interoperability of the ePHR have not been established to date (Halamka et al., 2005; Kaelber, Jha, Johnston, Middleton, & Bates, 2008; National Committee on Vital and Health Statistics, 2006; Reti, Feldman, & Safran, 2009). It is likely, however, that some patients/clients may have already adopted an ePHR, or have made the decision to create an ePHR. Those patients who do not have an ePHR may seek advice from the APN on how to select an ePHR.

The ePHRs generally assume one of three configurations (Tang, Ash, Bates, Overhage, & Sands, 2006). One configuration is the stand-alone ePHR. Examples include Google Health (Google, 2011), HealthVault (Microsoft, 2010), PHRs Today (H360 ventures, 2010), and ePHRs offered by health care plans. The choice of a stand-alone ePHR is solely within the control of the patient. Additionally, information entry and maintenance of stand-alone ePHRs are the responsibility of the patient or designated surrogate. It is the choice of the patient to grant access of his/her ePHR to family members, primary care providers, and other care providers. The limitations of a stand-alone ePHR include, first, the ongoing commitment necessary to maintain accuracy by ensuring that the ePHR is regularly reviewed and updated. Second, regardless of the diligence of the patient, providers may suspect the authenticity, accuracy, and completeness of the ePHR. Another available ePHR configuration is a hybrid model in which web access is provided for the patient to view a portion or all of the health data that is stored by his or her health provider's EHR. Additionally, the patient is able to update or enter selected information in the ePHR. Some providers are reluctant to enable data entry by the patient due to concerns about accuracy and the patient's health literacy.

The third ePHR option is one where patients are granted view-only web-based access to selected portions of their EHR record without the ability to amend or add data. The view-only and limited-data-entry EHR maintained by the individual's health care provider is often referred to as "patient portals" or porthole views into the patient's comprehensive health care record. The advantages of the view-only and limited-data-entry ePHR options include the availability to patients of more robust content as compared to the stand-alone ePHR, and the inclusion of data backup systems in the event of computer failure or natural disasters (Tang et al., 2006).

A variety of added services may be available with patient portals providers depending upon the services the provider is able to support. For example, patient portals may include one- or two-way email communication with the provider. Online appointment scheduling is a feature attractive to many patients. In addition to direct communication with the nurse or physician primary care provider, robust ePHRs may support communication with the pharmacies used by the patient, thus enabling a more comprehensive list of current medication therapies, and drug-drug or drug-allergy clinical decision support to the health provider. More comprehensive resources for ePHR assessment may be accessed at the Centers for Medicare and Medicaid Services (CMS, 2010) and the HIMSS websites (HIMSS, 2007, 2008).

Guiding Patient Discernment of Health Care Information on the Internet

As patients become increasingly adept in the use of information technology and the Internet, the APN may notice a change in the questions patients ask and in patients' knowledge about their health and in self-care. They may also seek advice about the veracity of various websites. The APN must equip the patient with information and tools that will guide them to make informed choices and feel confident that they are able to discern credible health care websites containing authentic, accurate, and useful information.

The proliferation of health and health care information available on the Internet is difficult to comprehend without initiating a search. To gain an appreciation of the pervasiveness of websites on the Internet that address health or health issues, you need only "Google" the term "health." A search conducted on April 3, 2011, disclosed nearly 2.4 trillion sites. The available information is overwhelming, and many patients need some assistance to determine the validity of the information present on these websites.

Over 80% of the American population searches the Internet for health and heath-related information (Fox, 2006). The authenticity of information patients find on the Internet is highly variable. Authenticity and accuracy concerns increase with the realization that the content of the Internet is not regulated. Consequently, health care information on the Internet should be carefully evaluated for accuracy and reliability prior to developing a level of confidence in the website content (Weber, Derrico, Yoon, & Sherwill-Navarro, 2009). Two important indicators of authenticity and accuracy of data on an Internet site are the source of the data and the date the site was last updated. Interestingly, 75% of people who search for health information on the Internet do not check the data source (e.g., author, credentials, affiliation, etc.) or the date that the website was last updated (Fox, 2006).

Health care websites vary in quality and accuracy of information, and patients seeking information are often vulnerable and not in the best position to discriminate among advice offered on health care websites. Researchers from the University of Florida (summarized in Exhibit 6.1), and

EXHIBIT 6.1
GATOR Website Assessment Criteria

Genuineness of information can be assessed by exploring the stated goals and purpose of the site. For example, Internet addressed ending with ".com" are commercial websites that are usually selling a product or service; information provided by commercial websites should be independently verified with a credible resource. Care should also be taken to examine logos and website names, which may be ingeniously designed to closely resemble highly trusted and credible sites.

Accuracy of the information is a second consideration. Look for a date to determine the last time the website was updated, which is often at the bottom of the page. Also look for indications of peer review. Consider seeking verification of information on other credible websites, particularly if the content is different from other credible sites.

Trustworthiness helps to ensure veracity and reliability of the information. Check for references from credible sources, the credentials of site authors,

(continued)

EXHIBIT 6.1 (*continued*)

and whether the authors are affiliated with established and respected organizations. The presence of contact information, such as telephone numbers and mail and email addresses, is another indication of trustworthiness.

Origin or source of the site content is another indicator of trustworthiness. In most cases authorship or sponsorship by a governmental (.gov in the United States), academic (.edu in the United States), research, or health care organization lends some assurance that the content is trustworthy.

Readability is an indicator of how well the average consumer will be able to read and understand the website content. Some sites are designed for use by health care professionals; patients need to understand that fact and seek sites that are created and maintained for use by the lay information consumer.

Adapted from Weber et al. (2009).

Michigan State University, (summarized in Table 6.2), provide guidelines to assist care providers and patients to more effectively evaluate website content on the Internet.

Proactive introduction of the subject of health care information available on the Internet and exploration of the patient's experiences when seeking such

TABLE 6.2
Telehealth Website Evaluation

Design	Links within the site or to other reference sources are recognizable and working. The site can be accessed from multiple browsers (e.g., Internet Explorer, Firefox, Safari, etc.).
Literacy	The site provides information that helps the user evaluate the credibility and trustworthiness of the site.
Information	Readability is demonstrated through the limited use of jargon; tables and charts are clear and well labeled; less common terminology is clearly explained.
Content	The site guides the reader's evaluation and understanding of the information presented, suggests questions they may direct to health care providers, directs users to other credible sources, etc. Advertising, if present, should be clearly distinguished from the content of the site.

Adapted from Whitten, P., Holtz, B., Cornacchione, J., & Wirth, C. (2011). An evaluation of telehealth websites for design, literacy, information and content. *Journal of Telemedicne and Telecare, 17,* 31–35.

information on the Internet may assist the APN to determine the patient's readiness for education about effective use of the Internet. Empowering patients with knowledge of how to evaluate the information on the Internet provides the opportunity for patients to openly discuss information they may have discovered, and may promote a greater sense of partnership and accountability for managing their health status. Once the APN understands the information and sources the patient is consulting, the APN can continue the patient's education by exploring when and where such new knowledge is complementary to the medical plan of care. Table 6.3 is a selection of current resources that can assist the APN to become more knowledgeable regarding Internet evaluation.

Ergonomics

Ergonomics is an applied science that defines the physical, cognitive, and organization requirements of the work environment. Ergonomics is an important consideration when designing tools or configuring the spaces in which practitioners work to promote effective and safe use of the tools (Harrison, Koppel, & Bar-Lev, 2007; Prensky, 2001). Ergonomics is an overarching principle embedded within informatics practice, is woven throughout each ANA nursing informatics practice standard, and recognizes the criticality of promoting a safe practice environment that minimizes the likelihood of injury (ANA, 2008). Incorporating ergonomic principles in the design of new environments or the retrofit of older work environments can reduce the risk of musculoskeletal injuries or other related injuries that often occur as the result of a poorly designed setting (Nielsen & Trinkoff, 2003).

TABLE 6.3
Additional Website Evaluation Resources

National Library of Medicine: "Evaluation Health Websites"	http://nnlm.gov/outreach/consumer/evalsite.html
Medical Library Association: "A User's Guide to Finding and Evaluating Health Information on the Web"	http://www.mlanet.org/resources/userguide.html
Toronto Public Library: "Website Evaluation Criteria for Health Sites"	http://chis.wikidot.com/sf-site-evaluation
Health on the Net Foundation: "The HON Code of Conduct for Medical and Health Web Sites"	http://www.hon.ch/HONcode/Conduct.html
MedLine Plus: "Evaluating Internet Health Information: A Tutorial From the National Library of Medicine"	http://www.nlm.nih.gov/medlineplus/webeval/webeval.html

An important ergonomic consideration is the computer workstation, which must be designed to enable the user to work with the computer without strain or risk of temporary or permanent injury. The duration of sustained use of a computer workstation and the number of people who will use a workstation influence the necessary space modifications that will promote safe use.

Expert resources are available to guide objective purchase decisions for furniture and equipment, and to guide workstation design. Occupational Safety and Health Administration (OSHA) and Columbia University each offer evidence-based checklists for evaluation of workstations and to guide purchasing decisions (Columbia University, 2008; OSHA, 2003). Researchers at Cornell University conducted an extensive investigation of ergonomics and computer workstations, and the University offers information and checklists to guide workstation set up procedures (Cornell University Ergonomics Web, 2010, 2011). The consultative services of certified ergonomic professionals are also available as another expert consideration when planning computer workstations (Board of Certification in Professional Ergonomics [BCPE]). Given the personal anguish, lost productivity, and costs associated with ergonomic work-related injuries, some organizations choose to have a certified professional ergonomics engineer as a permanent part of the staff.

Evaluation of Patient Care Equipment

Patient safety is a central consideration when decisions are made to purchase new or replacement equipment for use in the direct or indirect care of patients. A facet of effective equipment evaluation is assessment of the usability of that equipment. Usability addresses the design of devices with attention to how the device will be used, the ways in which people may abuse the device, the types of errors people could make while using the devices, and the outcomes people wish to achieve through use of the device (Norman, 2002; Phansalkar et al., 2010; Zhang, Johnson, Patel, Paige, & Kubose, 2003).

Usability is a dimension of human factors engineering; that is, it is information system design that focuses on the abilities and limitations of humans (Phillips, Repperger, & Reynolds, 2006) and biomedical informatics (e.g., application of informatics to improve the health of individuals, populations, the general public, and research) (Hersh, 2009) and that researches the interaction between people and technology. Human factors engineers focus their research on increasing knowledge about the capabilities and limitations of people. Human factors engineers then seek to design technology, processes, and systems that enhance the capabilities of people while compensating for their limitations. A good design process should make it easy to do the right thing and use the technology correctly while making it difficult to make mistakes, particularly mistakes that could harm the user or others.

A respected means of evaluating the usability of equipment of software is to examine and observe how the system or equipment is used. An APN can apply some of the basic principles of usability that are embodied in a process called heuristic testing, the principles of which are described in Table 6.4. These principles may prove useful to evaluate patient care technologies in APN practice. They are applicable when evaluating equipment, software, EHR designs, and similar situations. Heuristic evaluation principles are not difficult to apply and can support objective comparative information based on the usability characteristics of equipment, information systems, communication systems, and so forth.

TABLE 6.4

Usability Evaluation Using Heuristic Principles

Heuristic Principle	Example
1. Consistency and Standards	Does the application use color consistently and do the colors make sense? Are terms clear to the user and are they used consistently? Are buttons consistently used for the same purpose? Is there consistency in general layout between screens?
2. Visibility of the System State	Can the user tell when the system is working? Is the next action to be taken clear to the user?
3. Match Between the System and the World	Does use of the equipment match what the user would generally expect? Does pressing buttons or turning knobs result in expected outcomes? Does the user see what is expected?
4. Minimalist	Is the information present on the screen only what is needed to inform the user? Is superfluous information on the screen? Is there a logical and sequential level of detail and action?
5. Memory Load Is Minimized	Does the system require the user to rely on memory to use the equipment, or is the user appropriately prompted? Are examples for data entry expectations offered (e.g., YYYY/MM/DD or YY/MM/DD)? Does the system progress through a logical hierarchy?
6. Feedback That Is Informative	Does the system offer immediate and understandable feedback to user actions, particularly incorrect actions? Is the feedback specific, providing clear direction regarding the next step to be taken?

(continued)

TABLE 6.4 (*continued*)

Heuristic Principle	Example
7. Flexibility and Efficiency	Does the system support shortcuts for the experienced user? Are the information needs of the novice distinguished from those of the expert?
8. Good Error Messages	When the user makes an error, does the system provide a meaningful and understandable feedback message, enabling the user to learn from the error? Does the system avoid the use of error "codes" (e.g., "Error 147")? Are error messages polite and helpful (e.g., "fatal error," "illegal action")?
9. Preventing Error	Is the system designed to help the user avoid mistakes? Does the system prevent egregious errors? Are audible or pop-up messages present when the user is about to perform an incorrect action?
10. Clear Closure	Is it clear when a user is at the beginning, middle, or end of a task? Is it clear when a task, or required sequence of tasks, is completed?
11. Reversible Actions	Does the system allow the user to recover from mistakes? Does the system prevent serious errors? Does the system allow the user to explore the system and back out without consequences?
12. User Language	Does the system use language familiar to the user? Do the terms used by the system have a standard meaning?
13. User in Control	Is the user in control of the system? Does the user, not the system, initiate action?
14. Help and Documentation	Does the system provide context-sensitive help? Is the help embedded in the system? Is help available when needed?

Adapted from Graham et al. (2004); Norman (2002); Zhang et al. (2003).

Usability evaluation of patient care equipment is an important measure in reducing risk, increasing safety, and minimizing human error in the delivery of patient care. Cost, return on investment, functionality, and compatibility with the current clinical environment are important considerations in selection of patient care equipment from various vendor options. Equally important are the usability characteristics of each vendor's product. It is important to select equipment that is easy to use and that actively promotes the avoidance of error. The usability characteristics demonstrated by the equipment options under consideration for purchase should have at least equal weight with the other considerations in making the purchase decision. Zhang et al. (2003) suggest a rating scale to assist in assigning weights to the evaluation outcomes, which may be helpful when comparing the same equipment from different vendors.

A properly conducted heuristic evaluation is very unlikely to find no usability problems—the sophistication of human factors engineering has not attained that level of refinement to date. The primary intent of usability evaluation is to identify the product that is most appropriate for the target clinical environment. Additionally, usability evaluation will shed light on usability problems so that users can be informed of the risks and policies can be established to reduce and mitigate the identified risks.

SUMMARY

This discussion has established the role of an informatician and the criticality of developing and maintaining an ongoing partnership between nurse informaticians and APNs. This partnership can provide significant guidance to IT project design and implementation. The scope and variety of IT and how deeply it is embedded in practice and in personal and professional lives was briefly addressed. The national mandate for EHRs was discussed along with why EHR selection and implementation is such a central focus at this time.

The APN is in an excellent position to influence nursing practice and technology implementation. As a respected member of the health care team, the APN can identify the informatics competency needs of colleagues and staff and can influence understanding of the power of this essential skill, advocating for resources that will support skill building. The APN can empower patients to become more knowledgeable and involved in health maintenance, disease prevention, and management of chronic diseases through an understanding of the ePHR and can identify the patients in his/her practice that would benefit from the ePHR. Such understanding will inform the patient-teaching process and assist patients to discern authentic, accurate information on the Internet.

Also considered was the role of the APN in the influence of technology-driven patient care equipment purchase decisions though a constructive heuristic evaluation. The heuristic evaluation metrics presented can serve as important and objective criteria to evaluate patient care equipment. Design of computer workstations is important to avoid or minimize user injury. We established basic workflow design issues and, more importantly, directed readers to several evidence-based websites that described ergonomically appropriate computer design.

CASE STUDY

Anywhere Hospital has been using IV pumps for the past 20 years. Over the years, models from various vendors were researched and purchased. The complexity of the pumps increased with each subsequent purchasing cycle. The hospital currently maintains IV pumps from ten different vendors to meet the needs of critical care, trauma, anesthesiology, and the medical/surgical patient care units; five of these pumps are used on the medical/surgical units. The decision to purchase each brand of pump was based on new and enhanced patient safety features. The last model was purchased nearly five years ago, and each of the other brands received feature/function upgrades in the past four years.

While each of the pumps was purchased with the intent of increasing patient safety, Anywhere Hospital has also experienced unintended consequences. First, each pump has a different user interface, which has lengthened orientation for newly hired medical/surgical nurses. Second, the different interfaces have resulted in programming errors that have compromised patient safety. Because the demand for IV pumps is high, a nurse may be responsible for several IV pump brands in his or her patient care assignment. Third, the expense to inventory replacement parts and ensure biomedical engineering competency to repair the ten pump brands were not anticipated in the original cost of ownership projections.

Anywhere Hospital recently completed an analysis intended to "right size" the number and types of IV pumps necessary to provide safe, evidence-based IV therapy to the patients who entrust their lives to this health care organization. In addition to establishing the appropriate number and type of IV pumps that will meet the needs of the patient demographic mix cared for at Anywhere Hospital, several criteria were established to guide future decisions about information technology related to IV therapy.

- Anywhere Hospital recognized that a single pump brand/model most likely would not meet the needs of critical care, the Level I Trauma Center, anesthesiology, and the inpatient medical/surgical units. The primary goal was to identify a single pump brand to serve the medical/surgical clinical care areas of the hospital with the intent of reduced user interface confusion issues and reduced parts inventory and biomedical competency costs.
- A Request for Information (RFI) containing the requisite functions and safety features required by Anywhere Hospital would be issued to IV pump vendors.

(continued)

- Biomedical engineering, pharmacy, and nursing would collaborate to create multiple clinical scenarios to address usability (heuristic) in various clinical test situations in which an IV pump would be used, such as: 1) hang an initial bag of fluid; 2) initiate an IV bag with medication using the pump drug library; 3) titrate a medication drip; 4) titrate multiple drips through the same site/catheter; and 5) clear the pump for a new patient.
- All pump vendors that submit a successful response to the RFI will be invited to demonstrate their product in strict accordance with the clinical scenarios defined by Anywhere Hospital. Vendors with successful demonstrations will be required to leave a sample pump with Anywhere Hospital for 3 weeks to allow further usability testing, employing the heuristic evaluation principles.
- Two to three practicing nurses will be solicited to complete each usability (heuristic) clinical scenario after appropriate orientation to the use of the IV pump. Each scenario will be filmed to enable effective analysis of usability.
- Usability (heuristic) functionality will be scored in accordance with Zhang et al.'s methodology (Zhang et al., 2003).
- Purchase decisions will be heavily weighted by the scored usability (heuristic) test outcomes.

REFERENCES

American Medical Informatics Association. (2011). *Degree programs, certificate programs, fellowships, and short courses.* Retrieved from https://www.amia.org/informatics-academic-training-programs

American Medical Informatics Association Nursing Informatics Work Group. (2009, January 22). *Roles in nursing informatics.* Retrieved from https://www.amia.org/ni-wg/ni-wg-roles

American Nurses Association. (2008). *Nursing informatics: Scope and standards of practice.* Silver Springs, MD: Author.

Association of College and Research Libraries. (2000). *Information literacy competency standards for higher education* (p. 15). Chicago, IL: Author. Retrieved from http://www.ala.org/ala/mgrps/divs/acrl/standards/informationliteracycompetency.cfm

Board of Certification in Professional Ergonomics. Retrieved from http://www.bcpe.org/

Centers for Medicare & Medicaid Services. (2010, April 30). *Personal health record overview.* Retrieved from http://www.cms.gov/PerHealthRecords/

Centers for Medicare & Medicaid Services. (2011, February 25). *The medicare EHR incentive program.* Retrieved from http://www.cms.gov/EHRIncentivePrograms/#BOOKMARK1

Columbia University. (2008). *Ergonomic self-evaluation tool.* Retrieved from http://ehs columbia.edu/ErgoEvaluateTool.html

Cornell University Ergonomics Web. (2010). *Performance oriented ergonomic checklist for computer (VDT) workstations.* Retrieved from http://ergo.human.cornell.edu/CUVDTChecklist.html

Cornell University Ergonomics Web. (2011). *CUErgo*. Retrieved from http://ergo. human.cornell.edu/default.htm

Fox, S. (2006, October 29). *Online health search*. Retrieved from www.pewintervel.org/ Reports/2006

Google. (2011). *Google health(TM)*. Retrieved from https://www.google.com/accounts/ ServiceLogin?service=health&nui=1&continue=https://health.google.com/ health/p/&followup=https://health.google.com/health/p/&rm=hide

Graham, M. J., Kubose, T. K., Jordan, D., Zhang, J., Johnson, T. R., & Patel, V. L. (2004). Heuristic evaluation of infusion pumps: Implications for patient safety in Intensive Care Units. *International Journal of Medical Informatics, 73*(11–12), 771–779.

Greenes, R. A., & Shortliffe, E. H. (2009). Informatics in biomedicine and health care. *Academic Medicine, 84*(7), 818–820.

Gruber, D., Cummings, G. G., Leblanc, L., & Smith, D. L. (2009). Factors influencing outcomes of clinical information systems implementation: A systematic review. *CIN: Computers Informatics Nursing May/June, 27*(3), 151–163.

H360 ventures. (2010). *Personal health records: Resources to manage your health*. Retrieved from http://www.phrstoday.com/index.html

Halamka, J., Overhage, J. M., Ricciardi, L., Rishel, W., Shirky, C., & Diamond, C. (2005). Exchanging health information: Local distribution, national coordination. *Health Affairs, 24*(5), 1170–1179.

Harrison, M. I., Koppel, R., & Bar-Lev, S. (2007). Unintended consequences of information technologies in health care an interactive sociotechnical analysis. *Journal of the American Medical Informatics Association, 14*(5), 542–549. doi:10.1197/jamia. M2384

Health Information Management Systems Society (HIMSS) Nursing Informatics. (2011). *The role of the nurse informaticist*. Retrieved from http://www.himss. org/ASP/topics_FocusDynamic.asp?faid=243

Hersh, W. (2009). A stimulus to define informatics and health information technology. *BMC Medical Informatics and Decision Making, 9*(1), 24.

Health Information Management Systems Society. (2007, June 27). *HIMSS personal health records definition and position statement*. Retrieved from http://www. google.com/search?source=ig&hl=en&rlz=1G1GGLQ_ENUS310&=&q= Definition+and+Position+Statement&aq=f&aqi=&aql=&oq=#sclient=psy&hl= en&rlz=1G1GGLQ_ENUS310&source=hp&q=HIMSS+Personal+Health+Re cords+Definition+and+Position+Statemen&aq=f&aqi=&aql=&oq=&pbx=1& bav=on.2,or.r_gc.r_pw.&fp=6dcad21d8bd7a66e

Health Information Management Systems Society. (2008). *Electronic personal health records (ePHR) checklist*. Retrieved from http://www.google.com/search? source=ig&hl=en&rlz=1G1GGLQ_ENUS310&=&q=Definition+and+Position+ Statement&aq=f&aqi=&aql=&oq=#sclient=psy&hl=en&rlz=1G1GGLQ_ENUS 310&q=HIMSS+electronic+Personal+Health+Records+checklist&aq=o&aqi=& aql=&oq=&pbx=1&bav=on.2,or.r_gc.r_pw.&fp=8287763aa926b759

Health Information Management Systems Society Analytics. (2010). *Essentials of the U.S. Hospital IT Market*. Retrieved from http://www.himssanalytics.org/docs/ Essentials/5thEditionEssentialsEMRAM.pdf

Hilbert, M., & Lopez, P. (2011). The world's technological capacity to store, communicate, and compute information. *Science, 331*. doi:10.1126/science.1200970

Kaelber, D. C., Jha, A. K., Johnston, D., Middleton, B., & Bates, D. W. (2008). A research agenda for personal health records (PHRs). *JAMIA, 15*(6), 729–736.

Koppel, R., Wetterneck, T., Telles, J. L., & Karsh, B.-T. (2008). Workarounds to barcode medication administration systems: Their occurrences, causes, and threats to patient safety. *Journal of the American Medical Informatics Association, 15*(4), 408–423. doi:10.1197/jamia.M2616

Linden Resarch Inc. (2011). *Second life.* Retrieved from http://secondlife.com/

McLane, S., & Turley, J. P. (2011). Informaticians: How they may benefit your healthcare organization. *Journal of Nursing Administration, 41*(1), 29–35.

Microsoft. (2010). *HealthVault.* Retrieved from http://www.healthvault. com/personal/index.aspx?WT.mc_id=M10011232&WT.ad=text:: Personal_Medical_Record::GoogSrch::HvPHp::Goo&WT.srch=1&WT.seg_1= personal%20medical%20records&rmproc=true

National Committee on Vital and Health Statistics. (2006, February 6). *Personal health records and personal health record systems.* Retrieved from http://www. google.com/search?source=ig&hl=en&rlz=1G1GGLQ_ENUS310&=&q= 28%29%09National+Committee+on+Vital+and+Health+Statistics.+%28200 6%29.+Personal+health+records+and+personal+health+record+systems& aq=f&aqi=&aql=&oq=

Nielsen, K. R. M., & Trinkoff, A. S. R. N. F. (2003). Applying ergonomics to nurse computer workstations: Review and recommendations. *CIN: Computers Informatics Nursing May/June, 21*(3), 150–157.

Norman, D. A. (2002). *The design of everyday things.* New York, NY: Basic Books.

Obama, B. (2009, February 9). Obama's prime-time press briefing. *The New York Times.* Retrieved from http://www.nytimes.com/2009/02/09/us/politics/ 09text-obama.html?pagewanted=1&_r=1

Occupational Safety and Health Administration. (2003, August). *Computer workstations.* Retrieved from http://www.osha.gov/SLTC/etools/computer-workstations/

Office of the National Coordinator for Health Information Technology. (2011, March 24). *Federal health information technology strategic plan 2011–2015.* Retrieved from http://healthit.hhs.gov/portal/server.pt/document/954074/ federal_hit_strategic_plan_public_comment_period

Phansalkar, S., Edworthy, J., Hellier, E., Seger, D. L., Schedlbauer, A., Avery, A. J., & Bates, D. W. (2010). A review of human factors principles for the design and implementation of medication safety alerts in clinical information systems. *JAMIA, 17*(5), 493–501. doi:10.1136/jamia.2010.005264

Phillips, C. A., Repperger, D. W., & Reynolds, D. B. (2006). *Human factors engineering.* Hoboken, NJ: John Wiley & Sons.

Prensky, M. (2001). Digital natives, digital immigrants, part I. *On the Horizon, 9*(5).

Reti, S. R., Feldman, H. J., & Safran, C. (2009). Governance for personal health records. *Journal of the American Medical Informatics Association, 16*(1), 14–17.

Staggers, N., Gassert, C. A., & Curran, C. (2001). Informatics competencies for nurses at four levels of practice. *Journal of Nursing Education, 40*(7), 303–316.

Tang, P. C., Ash, J. S., Bates, D. W., Overhage, J. M., & Sands, D. Z. (2006). Personal health records: Definitions, benefits, and strategies for overcoming barriers to adoption. *Journal of American Medical Informatics Association, 13*(2), 121–126.

Technology Informatics Guiding Education Reform. (2007). *Evidence and informatics transforming nursing: 3-year action steps toward a 10-year vision.* Retrieved from http:// www.tigersummit.com/Summit.html

Technology Informatics Guiding Education Reform. (2009). *Collaborating to integrate evidence and informatics into nursing practice and education: An executive summary.* Retrieved from http://www.tigersummit.com/9_Collaboratives.html

Vastag, B. (2011, February 10). *Exabytes: Documenting the 'digital age' and huge growth in computing capacity.* Retrieved from http://www.washingtonpost.com/wp-dyn/content/article/2011/02/10/AR2011021004916.html?sid=ST2011021100514

Weber, B. A., Derrico, D. J., Yoon, S. L., & Sherwill-Navarro, P. (2009). Educating patients to evaluate web-based health care information: The GATOR approach to healthy surfing. *Journal of Clinical Nursing, 19,* 1371–1377.

Whitten, P., Holtz, B., Cornacchione, J., & Wirth, C. (2011). An evaluation of telehealth websites for design, literacy, information and content. *Journal of Telemedicne and Telecare, 17,* 31–35.

Zhang, J., Johnson, T. R., Patel, V. L., Paige, D. L., & Kubose, T. (2003). Using usability heuristics to evaluate patient safety of medical devices. *Journal of Biomedical Informatics, 36*(1–2), 23–30.

SEVEN

Evaluation of Patient Care Standards, Guidelines, and Protocols

Ronda G. Hughes

"Unless we are making progress in our nursing every year, every month, every week, take my word for it we are going back."

Florence Nightingale

INTRODUCTION

APNs are often called upon to evaluate individual and population health based on achievement of health outcomes that represent quality indicators of health and care. This chapter examines the evaluation of patient care based on accepted standards and guidelines. The Institute of Medicine's *Roundtable on Evidence-Based Medicine* (2008) set a goal that "by 2020, ninety percent of clinical decisions should be supported by accurate, timely, and up-to-date clinical information that reflects the best available evidence." That is a lofty goal as it has been estimated that about 20% of clinical decisions are evidence based (McGlynn et al., 2003). Of the more than $2 trillion annually invested in health care, less than 0.1% is devoted to evaluating the relative effectiveness of the various diagnostics, procedures, devices, pharmaceuticals, and other interventions in clinical practice (Academy Health, 2005; Moses, Dorsey, Matheson, & Their, 2005). In order to appreciate what these standards, guidelines, and protocols represent, a review of the background and development of each will be explored so that the APN can critically review these entities before adoption or translation into practice.

The delivery and quality of health care services vary. Researchers continue to find variation associated with practice patterns, socio-demographics of populations, and geographic location. Health care leaders, managers, policy makers and practitioners have been concerned about this variation and have been actively involved in various strategies to bring and drive health care toward high quality consistency. Many of these efforts have involved developing, implementing, and enforcing standards, guidelines, and protocols as part of evidence-based practices.

TYPES OF RESEARCH INFLUENCING PATIENT CARE

Research is evaluated through various mechanisms and can support or refute current or proposed standards, guidelines, and protocols. There are several major types of research that are used to influence patient care decisions. Randomized controlled trials (RCTs) is a form of clinical trial or experimental type of research that is commonly used to test the safety and efficacy or effectiveness of health care services (e.g., a type of surgical procedure) and is held by many to be the "gold standard." Considering the scope and depth of clinical and health care research and the cost of conducting a RCT, other forms of research can also be successfully used to inform practice. For example, descriptive research provides data and characteristics about a population or phenomenon, but does not describe what factors may have caused a situation; for instance, the number of people within a specific population that have been diagnosed and are being managed for diabetes mellitus. There is also research that statistically assesses the relationship (or correlation) between two or more random variables. For example, determining a predictive relationship between the flu season and demand for clinician visits or emergency department utilization may suggest the numbers of people affected and the severity of symptoms. Another type of research draws a sample from a larger population and makes a distinction between those with selected risk factors and those without it. These two cohorts are followed over a period of time to determine the frequency and timing during which the outcomes of interest occur. Additionally, qualitative research provides insight into the social processes, subcultures, experiences, and perceptions of individuals and populations that are generally not detectible through databases or other sources of information. Together the different types of research can be used to inform the development, testing, and implementation of standards, guidelines, and protocols.

The information or research supporting practice and changes in how care is delivered varies. This information can range from a *recommendation*, a suggestion for practice that is not necessarily approved by expert groups, to a guideline that was the product of intensive research evidence and consensus among experts. The following section provides definitions and a brief discussion of a number of terms as a basis for further discussion.

Basic Concepts

The following includes selected basic concepts that are foundational for understanding standards, guidelines, and protocols. They include indicators, standards, guidelines, protocols, best practices, and evidence-based practice.

Indicators

Indicators are visible signs of whether or not an intervention or program is achieving the expected outcomes or progressing in the intended direction (Robert Wood Johnson Foundation, 2004). An indicator is a measurable surrogate (e.g., number or percentage) that is considered representative of an outcome and that can be tracked to determine if there is an increase, decrease, or an improvement or deterioration in the outcome. *Quality indicators* are measures of health care quality that make use of readily available hospital administrative data.

Standards

Standards are considered to be the level and type of care expected. They reflect a desired and achievable level of performance against which actual performance can be compared. The main purpose of standards is to promote, guide, and direct practice (College of Registered Nurses of Nova Scotia, 2004). According to the Healthcare Information and Management Systems Society (HIMSS), a standard is "a document established by consensus and approved by a recognized body, or is accepted as a de facto standard by the industry" (HIMSS, 2010, p. 113). Standards of care are developed over time or are the result of findings from clinical and health care research, and can vary by state or community (Emanuel, 1997).

In legal terms, a standard of care is used as the benchmark against how a clinician practices. If, for example, the U.S. Department of Health and Human Services declares a treatment procedure as not safe and effective, then the practitioners who employ such treatment procedures can be deemed as not meeting the professionally recognized standards of health care. Professionally recognized standards are applicable to practitioners providing care and are recognized by the professional peers of a clinician/ clinical group. However, this does not mean that all other treatments meet the professionally recognized standards of care. In a malpractice lawsuit, the clinician's lawyer will want to prove that the clinician's actions were aligned with the standard of care. The plaintiff's lawyer will want to show how the clinician violated the accepted standard of care and was therefore negligent (Moffett & Moore, 2011).

All industries have some form of standard by which quality is judged. According to the American Nurses Association (ANA), a standard is an "authoritative statement enunciated and promulgated by the profession by which the quality of practice, service, or education can be judged" (ANA, 2004, p. 115). In another publication the ANA describes standards as authoritative statements by which the nursing profession describes the responsibilities for which its practitioners are accountable. Standards reflect the values and priorities of the profession and provide direction for professional nursing practice and a framework for the evaluation of practice. Standards also define the nursing profession's accountability to the public and the outcomes for which registered nurses are responsible (ANA, 2010).

For nurses, there are standards of care promulgated by professional nursing organizations. For example, the ANA promotes nursing excellence through standards, a code of ethics, and credentialing. The ANA standards describe the responsibilities for which its practitioners are accountable, reflect the values and priorities of the profession, and provide direction for professional nursing practice and a framework for the evaluation of this practice. These standards also define the nursing profession's accountability to the public and the outcomes for which registered nurses are responsible.

The ANA Standards of Professional Performance describe a competent level of behavior for professional nurses, including activities related to quality of care, performance appraisal, education, collegiality, ethics, collaboration, research, and resource utilization. These standards serve as guidelines for accountability and are designed to ensure that patients receive high-quality care. The standards specifically guide nurses to know exactly what is necessary to provide quality nursing care, and the measures that can be used to determine whether the care meets the standards. Of these standards, two in particular will be discussed for illustrative purposes.

First, the *quality of practice* requires that the registered nurse systematically enhances the quality and effectiveness of nursing practice (ANA, 2010). The measurement criteria are:

1. Demonstrates quality by documenting the application of the nursing process in a responsible, accountable, and ethical manner.
2. Uses quality improvement activities to initiate changes in nursing practice and health care delivery system.
3. Uses creativity and innovation to improve nursing care delivery.
4. Incorporates new knowledge to initiate changes in nursing practice if desired outcomes are not achieved.
5. Participates in quality improvement activities (ANA, 2004, 2010).

Second, the *research standard* is defined as "the nurse integrates research findings in practice" (ANA, 2010). This is measured with the following criteria:

1. Utilize best available evidence including research findings to guide practice decisions.

2. Participates in research activities as appropriate to the nurse's education and position such as the following:
   a. Identifying clinical problems suitable for nursing research
   b. Participating in data collection
   c. Participating in a unit, organization, or community research committee
   d. Sharing research activities with others conducting research
   e. Critiquing research for application to practice
   f. Uses research findings in the development of policies, procedures, and practice guidelines for patient care
   g. Incorporates research as a basis for learning. (ANA, 2004, 2010)

Nurses demonstrate the standards of care for professional nursing through the nursing process. This involves assessment, diagnosis, outcome identification, planning, implementation, and evaluation. The nursing process is the foundation of clinical decision making and encompasses all significant actions taken by nurses in providing care to all patients. Accountability for one's professional practice rests with the individual nurse. The standards of care in the ANA's (2004, 2010) *Nursing: Scopes and Standards of Practice* describe a competent level of nursing care, which are demonstrated through the nursing process. Standards of care are also important if a legal dispute arises over whether a nurse practiced appropriately in a particular case.

Guidelines

Guidelines can be defined generically or specifically to clinical practice. A *guideline* is a description that clarifies what should be done and how it should be done to achieve the given objectives (HIMSS, 2010, p. 55). Guidelines are developed to standardized care based on what is considered to be the best available evidence and information. When possible, guidelines are based on research. *Clinical practice guidelines* are a set of systematically developed statements, usually based on scientific evidence, to assist practitioners and patient decision makers about appropriate health care for specific clinical circumstances (HIMSS, 2010, p. 21). Clinical practice guidelines are produced by government agencies, health care systems, professional organizations, and specialty centers.

There are many steps in developing guidelines, each of which can be vulnerable to bias or error. This may result in the misuse or misinterpretation of research evidence and, therefore, its translation into a clinical practice guideline. There are various strategies in developing guidelines, but there is no universal standard mechanism to ensure that each published guideline was developed in the best way possible (Guyatt et al., 2006). Generally, the process begins with identifying and refining the subject area of a possible guideline. Next, a group (optimally, versus an individual) engages stakeholders and identifies and assesses the evidence. This group then summarizes, categorizes, and critically evaluates available evidence to determine the quality and strength of the evidence. This evaluation of the evidence is then translated into a clinical practice guideline. The guideline is then reviewed by experts in the field and key stakeholders. After a guideline is published, it should be updated frequently to reflect new research and knowledge when available.

Acknowledging that clinical guidelines were becoming more a part of clinical practice, Woolf, Grol, Hutchinson, Eccles, and Grimshaw (1999) discussed use of guidelines in terms of the benefits from encouraging the use of interventions proven to be successful and informing decision making, and the harms of misleading decision makers because the evidence informing the guideline was limited, misinterpreted, or biased, which may have incorrectly influenced the recommendation(s). These and many other concerns have been raised about guidelines. In a recent report, the Institute of Medicine (IOM) set forth eight standards for clinical practice guidelines: 1) establishing transparency; 2) management of conflict of interest; 3) guideline development group composition; 4) clinical practice guideline-systematic review intersection; 5) establishing evidence foundations for and rating strength; 6) articulation of recommendations; 7) external review; and 8) updating (IOM, 2011a, 2011b). As such, APNs must be careful in implementing/adapting clinical guidelines in that for many topics/situations, there are a multitude of guidelines. These guidelines may not concur with each other and most likely were developed using different processes and different sources of evidence. To address these concerns, APNs must carefully consider each guideline and evaluate the best match to their practice and patient population.

Protocols

A clinical *protocol* is a set of rules defining a standardized treatment program or behavior in specific circumstances (HIMSS, 2010, p. 21). A protocol is a detailed guide for approaching a clinical problem and is designed to address a specific practice situation. It is often agency specific. For example, a check list for pressure ulcer prevention including assessment steps and timeline for turning and repositioning patients might be look very different from agency to agency because they were developed specifically for each agency.

Protocols exist to reduce variation in care for a specific patient population. They are generally to be adhered to in practice, particularly when the recommended actions have been scientifically studied and experts in the field have considered and advised on their application. Clinical protocols are defined as standards of care that define specific care actions that should be given to a defined patient population. Many specify how, when, and by whom a specific action should be performed. Some clinical protocols present a comprehensive plan of care, such as perioperative and postoperative care for elderly patients undergoing joint replacement surgery, whereas other protocols address just one aspect of care such as prophylactic antibiotics administration before joint replacement surgery.

Best Practices

A *best practice* describes a process or technique for which application in practice results in improved patient and/or organizational outcomes. A best practice is something that an individual, group, or organization can apply to practice to perform significantly better than other individual, groups, or organizations. From a non-scientific perspective, best practices can also be defined as the most efficient (i.e., least amount of effort) and most effective (i.e., best results) way of accomplishing a task, based on replicable procedures that have proven themselves over time for large numbers of people. A best practice is applicable to particular condition or circumstance and may have to be modified or adapted for similar circumstances.

Various organizations, professional associations, and many others publish "best practices" to inform clinical decision making. Generally, best practices are accepted, informally standardized techniques, methods, or processes that have been proven over time to accomplish given tasks. These practices are commonly used, but are generally based on no specific formal methodology. It is assumed that if done right, using best practices will achieve a desired outcome across organizations that can be delivered more effectively and consistently.

An APN searching for best practices for any given question will usually begin with a review of the literature so that research and other sources of evidence inform best practices. It rests upon the APN to evaluate the literature to determine the basis and strength of a possible intervention based on the source, reliability, and quality of the information and the methods used to define the "best practice." Although meta-analysis is considered the highest level of research evidence, clinical questions in practice do not always have supportive research of such quantity and quality to provide this level of evidence. Therefore, the APN must review what literature is available to make a judgment about what might be potentially a better or best practice in a given situation.

Evidence-Based Practice

Evidence-based practice is a problem-solving approach to clinical decision making within a health care organization that integrates the best available research evidence with the best available experiential (patient and practitioner) evidence. Both internal and external influences on practice are considered, and critical thinking in the judicious application of evidence is considered (Newhouse, Dearholt, Poe, Pugh, & White, 2007). Evidence-based practice is based on research evidence about the effectiveness of interventions that are used to guide decision making about patient care. It relies on a ranking of the multiple research studies that critically differentiates the most to the least reliable research findings. This is important because individual research findings can be misleading for a variety of reasons ranging from a poor study design to a small sample size that is not generalizable (Sackett et al., 2000).

Even when evidence is available, many research studies have identified significant gaps between actual practice and the best possible practice. Part of this gap has been because of the lack of research evidence to inform and standardize practice to achieve predictable outcomes. Another part of this gap reflects the view that evidence-based practice discounts individual clinical skills and patient preferences (Closs & Cheater, 1999). Although in many instances there is no research evidence, the aim of evidence-based practice is to integrate current best evidence from research with clinical policy and practice. In doing so, clinical decision making can be based on evidence-informed tools of what works to improve performance, narrow the gap between practice and research, and improve patient outcomes (Bates et al., 2003).

To apply evidence-based practices, APNs need to implement the best interventions and practices that are informed by the best evidence. From the perspectives of quality and safety, evidence-based practice is considered the gold standard of care. Evidence-based practice can "raise the bar" within clinical practice and achieve more predicable patient outcomes.

MAJOR INFLUENCES ON SHAPING AND EVALUATING HEALTH CARE

The Institute of Medicine

The Institute of Medicine (IOM) is a non-profit, private organization, the purpose of which is to provide national advice on issues relating to biomedical science, medicine, and health to improve health care. It relies on a volunteer workforce of scientists and other experts operating under a rigorous, formal peer-review system. The IOM strives to provide unbiased, evidence-based, and authoritative information and advice concerning health and science policy issues. With its release of *To Err Is Human* (Kohn, Corrigan, & Donaldson, 2000), the IOM began a series of reports on improving quality and safety of health care. These reports have been instrumental in influencing quality and safety imperatives, national policy, and reimbursement.

In *Crossing the Quality Chasm: A New Health System for the 21st Century* (IOM, 2001), the IOM set forth six aims for health care improvement. These aims of safety, effective, timely, patient-centered, efficient, and equitable treatment have become a standard throughout health care. In terms of other standards, the IOM also asserted that chronic diseases were best managed when a "protocol or plan that provides an explicit statement of what needs to be done for patients, at what intervals, and by whom, and that considers the needs of all patients with specific clinical features and how their needs can be met" (IOM, 2001, p. 94).

The report, *Keeping Patient Safe: Transforming the Work Environment of Nurses*, emphasized the evidence for nursing and set forth policy recommendations primarily regarding nurse staffing. The IOM focused its recommendations on improving patient safety through strategies that would improve the work environment for nurses. Among the many recommendations were adequate staffing, organizational support for ongoing learning, and decision support, using mechanisms that promote interdisciplinary collaboration, and implementing a work design that promotes safety. While important for patients, practitioners, and organizations, the challenge is acting upon these recommendations in lieu of sufficient evidence for specific interventions that can optimize outcomes across organizations. The IOM (2004a) recommended minimal staffing levels for registered nurses and licensed nurses in nursing homes, but because there was insufficient evidence, the IOM could not recommend minimal staffing levels for acute care settings/hospitals.

In *Patient Safety: Achieving a New Standard for Care*, the IOM set forth recommendations to improve patient safety. One of the major recommendations was to better manage health information technology and data systems to enable patient safety as a standard across care delivery sites. Health information technology and data systems are needed to inform care decisions and support patient safety. To operationalize these recommendations, the IOM specified the need for common data standards for information sharing and utilization (IOM, 2004b).

The IOM has also addressed issues relating to evidence and how it should be used. In *Knowing What Works in Health Care: A Roadmap for the Nation*, the IOM recommended government oversight of the production of information for comparative effectiveness and to set forth high priority topics for systematic reviews of clinical effectiveness (IOM, 2008). The IOM also recommended that methodological standards and a common language for characterizing the strength of the evidence be developed for systematic reviews (IOM, 2008). Since these recommendations were made, an oversight committee has been developed and millions of dollars have been allocated by the federal government for comparative effectiveness research under the health care reform law passed in March 2010.

In *Knowing What Works in Health Care: Standards for Systematic Reviews*, the IOM responded to a directive from Congress to develop standards for conducting systematic reviews of the comparative effectiveness of medical and surgical interventions. These standards are intended to ensure that systematic reviews will be objective, transparent, and scientifically valid. In this report, the IOM recommended standards for the entire systematic review process, making specific recommendations on finding and assessing individual studies, synthesizing the body of evidence, and reporting systematic reviews.

The Joint Commission

Formerly the Joint Commission on Accreditation of Healthcare Organizations (JCAHO), the Joint Commission (JC) is a private, non-profit organization that provides elective accreditation of over 19,000 health care organizations and programs in the United States. The JC seeks to improve health care by encouraging and evaluating health care organizations. Organizations can receive accreditation only when they demonstrate achievement of specific performance standards. The United States government recognizes JC accreditation as a condition for Medicare and Medicaid reimbursement and licensure (JC, 2008).

The JC's standards for acute care hospital set the precedent for standards in other settings, and are even quoted in the judgments of some civil malpractice cases. When there are changes in the JC's standards, they are generally consistent with changes in federal policy and precedent-setting court cases, as well as changes in national concerns (e.g., sentinel events) or major reports (e.g., the IOM report, *To Err Is Human*).

Consistent with its stated mission of "improving health care for the public," the JC has set forth standards, goals, and measures to promote improvements in patient safety. To receive accreditation, health care organizations need to achieve a series of standards that represent high quality care. The JC's National Patient Safety Goal (NPSG) highlights problematic areas in health care and describes available evidence and expert-based solutions to these problems, if they exist (JC, 2011a). The NPSGs have become a critical method by which the JC promotes and enforces major changes in patient safety. The JC also sets forth quality improvement measures, and works with the Centers for Medicare and Medicaid Services on common national hospital performance measures (JC, 2011b).

In 1990, the then JCAHO dropped their Managed Care Accreditation Program and turned their accredited managed care organizations over to the National Committee for Quality Assurance (NCQA). The NCQA's first standards for managed care were published in 1991, and have been revised about every two years since then. The NCQA works with managed care organizations, health care purchasers, state regulators, and consumers to develop standards and performance measures that are intended to evaluate the structure and functions of medical and quality management systems in managed care organizations (see http://www.ncqa.org/tabid/59/default. aspx for information on the Health Plan Employer Data Information Set).

Centers for Medicare and Medicaid Services

As part of the U.S. Department of Health and Human Services (HHS), the Centers for Medicare and Medicaid Services (CMS), previously knows at the Health Care Financing Administration, administers the Medicare program and works in partnership with state governments to administer Medicaid, the State Children's Health Insurance Program (SCHIP), and health insurance portability standards. CMS is also responsible for the administrative simplification standards from the Health Insurance Portability and Accountability Act of 1996 (HIPAA), quality standards in long-term care facilities, and clinical laboratory quality standards under the Clinical Laboratory Improvement Amendments (see www.cms.gov). Throughout its programs and responsibilities, the CMS exerts tremendous influence on practice standards by setting forth reimbursement policies for covered services and by developing, interpreting, implementing, and evaluating policies for professional standards review, related peer review, utilization review, and utilization control programs. Hospitals receiving Medicare and Medicaid reimbursement must meet specific requirements and conditions established by the CMS to receive reimbursement for providing services to Medicare and Medicaid beneficiaries. These conditions include patients' rights, quality assessment, performance improvement, and utilization review.

Agency for Healthcare Research and Quality

Formerly the Agency for Healthcare Policy and Research, the Agency for Healthcare Research and Quality (AHRQ) is also part of the HHS. The mission of AHRQ is to improve the quality, safety, efficiency, and effectiveness of health care for all Americans, which helps the HHS achieve its strategic goals: to improve the safety, quality, affordability, and accessibility of health care; to promote public health and protection, disease prevention, and emergency preparedness; to promote the economic and social well-being of individuals, families, and communities; and to advance scientific and biomedical research and development related to health and human services. The AHRQ facilitates the development of evidence through research grants and evidence-based research syntheses through its evidence-based practice centers (www.ahrq.gov/clinic/epc). Research funded by the AHRQ helps individuals make more informed decisions and helps improve the quality of health care services. With quality and patient safety indicators (www.qualityindicators.ahrq.gov), the AHRQ works with organizations, such as the National Quality Forum, to set forth evidence-based indicators of quality.

After the AHRQ's "near death experience" from Congress in 1995 over its release of guidelines for back surgery, it turned the business of developing guidelines to non-governmental organizations including professional organizations. While not directly involved in guideline development, an important repository of guidelines covering a variety of topics is maintained by the AHRQ (which can be found at www.guidelines.gov).

HOW STANDARDS, GUIDELINES, AND PROTOCOLS ARE DEVELOPED

There are significant variations and several major forces in defining practice guidelines and protocols. Researchers apply various science-based methodologies to develop the research that can serve as the evidence. Experts and practitioners weigh in with their opinions based on personal experience and continue the tradition through education and reinforcement in practice settings. National health policy leaders and insurers influence minimal standards of care and define what services will be reimbursed and where. The public influences what type of care is expected through public opinion, the new media, and publications. Patients and their families influence what care is provided through preferences and interactions with practitioners. When standards, guidelines, and protocols are developed, many forces come together. For example, clinical, administrative, and academic experts developed the standards of nursing practice (ANA, 2004, 2010).

Process of Developing Standards, Guidelines, and Protocols

In many instances, practice guidelines are used to convey a synthesis of the strengths and weaknesses of the research and its practice implications, and to provide a basis to improve care quality by reducing practice variations (Baker, 2001). It can take 5 years for published guidelines to be adopted into routine practice (Lomas, Sisk, & Stocking, 1993). Even when guidelines exist and are broadly accepted, they are often not used in practice (Feder, Eccles, Grol, Griffiths, & Grimshaw, 1999).

The IOM has asserted that clinical guidelines should be used to guide health care decisions by practitioners and patients (Field & Lohr, 1990). Yet the strength of the guideline and its applicability to practice is dependent upon appropriate interpretation of the research evidence that is developed using formal methods. These methods should include identification of the area or areas of practice where a guideline could be helpful, synthesis of relevant research evidence, review by a guideline development group, and external review of the recommendations for the guidelines (Eccles & Grimshaw, 2004; Shekelle, Woolf, Eccles, & Grimshaw, 1999).

Research Evidence

Research tests innovations in laboratories and in practice. The millions of dollars that many public and private organizations invest in research provide hope that health care services can be improved. The challenge is that evidence developed through research has a tendency to "sit" in research journals and not be used in practice. It can take approximately 17 years for research to become part of practice (Balas & Boren, 2002).

Unfortunately, there is often a disconnect between research efforts and clinical practice. To improve the use of research in practice, the research evidence must be synthesized because only rarely should findings from one research project be implemented into practice. Conclusions from synthesized research can then be used to develop clinical practice recommendations and policy. It is then up to organizational leaders and practitioners to apply the recommendations and policy in the right setting, at the right time, and in the right manner. These steps help form a link between research and practice.

Synthesizing and Grading the Evidence

Findings from research are published primarily in peer-reviewed research journals. Various strategies have been developed to assess the quality of the research evidence. Practitioners can find research syntheses from groups, such as evidence-based practice centers (see www.ahrq.gov/clinic/epc), the Cochrane Collaboratives (see www.cochrane.org), the peer-reviewed literature, and information services that systematically review and evaluate the literature for specified topics and questions (AHRQ, 2010).

There are several challenges for both those doing the reviews and those reading the findings. First, these reviews and critical evaluations of research findings are dependent upon the research that has been completed, which may have only some bearing on the questions at hand. Second, many of the systematic reviews and efforts to inform guidelines hold randomized clinical trials (RCTs) as the gold standard, whereas the majority of the knowledge gaps in clinical practice cannot be adequately addressed by RCTs. And third, how the research is synthesized and evaluated is dependent upon the reviewers, the inclusion and exclusion criteria, and the criteria used to evaluate the research (Timmermans & Berg, 2003).

Another mechanism to locate and utilize synthesized research findings by integrating them into practice is through health information technology, such as clinical decision support systems that are sometimes integrated into electronic medical records. Optimally, electronic decision support systems enhance clinical practice and decision making with real-time information, but they must keep current with changes in evidence and clinical practice (Bates et al., 2003).

In practice, with particular patients, practitioners can search various sources of evidence. To effectively search evidence-based practice resources, it is helpful to decide what details are important to the clinical question at hand so that the right questions can be asked. According to Sackett and colleagues (2000), a well-built clinical question includes the following components:

- The patient's disorder or disease
- The intervention or finding under review
- A comparison intervention (if applicable—not always present)
- The outcome

The acronym PICOT, from these four components, has been used to assist in remembering the steps: P, patient/population or problem; I, intervention or issue of interest; C, comparison intervention or issue of interest; O, outcome(s) of interest; and the additional T, time it takes for the intervention to achieve the outcome(s) (Stillwell, Fineout-Overhold, Melynk, & Williamson, 2010).

Several strategies have been developed to evaluate the quality of evidence and the strength of practice recommendations. The strategies have different approaches to evaluating the evidence and have strengths and limitations according to the criteria used to evaluate the evidence and the subjectivity of the reviewers using a specific strategy (Atkins et al., 2004). The U.S. Preventive Services Task Force (USPSTF) developed a system (Table 7.1) to stratify evidence by quality for purposes of ranking evidence concerning the effectiveness of treatments or screening (USPSTF, 2008).

In evaluating the research evidence, the USPSTF makes recommendations for a clinical service based on a balance of risk versus benefit and the level of evidence on which the recommendation can be based. The USPSTF used the following levels to reflect the strength of the recommendation for clinical practice:

- Level A: Good scientific evidence suggests that the benefits of the clinical service substantially outweigh the potential risks. Clinicians should discuss the service with eligible patients.
- Level B: At least fair scientific evidence suggests that the benefits of the clinical service outweigh the potential risks. Clinicians should discuss the service with eligible patients.
- Level C: At least fair scientific evidence suggests that there are benefits provided by the clinical service, but the balance between benefits and risks are too close for making general recommendations. Clinicians need not offer it unless there are individual considerations.
- Level D: At least fair scientific evidence suggests that the risks of the clinical service outweigh potential benefits. Clinicians should not routinely offer the service to asymptomatic patients.

TABLE 7.1
U.S. Preventive Services Task Force Evidence Grading System

High	The available evidence usually includes consistent results from well-designed, well-conducted studies in representative primary care populations. These studies assess the effects of the preventive service on health outcomes. This conclusion is therefore unlikely to be strongly affected by the results of future studies.
Moderate	The available evidence is sufficient to determine the effects of the preventive service on health outcomes, but confidence in the estimate is constrained by such factors as: • The number, size, or quality of individual studies • Inconsistency of findings across individual studies • Limited generalizability of findings to routine primary care practice • Lack of coherence in the chain of evidence As more information becomes available, the magnitude or direction of the observed effect could change, and this change may be large enough to alter the conclusion.
Low	The available evidence is insufficient to assess effects on health outcomes. Evidence is insufficient because of: • The limited number or size of studies • Important flaws in study design or methods • Inconsistency of findings across individual studies • Gaps in the chain of evidence • Findings not generalizable to routine primary care practice • Lack of information on important health outcomes More information may allow estimation of effects on health outcomes.

■ Level I (Insufficient): Scientific evidence is lacking, of poor quality, or conflicting, such that the risk versus benefit balance cannot be assessed. Clinicians should help patients understand the uncertainty surrounding the clinical service. (USPSTF, 2008)

Another system for rating the hierarchy of evidence is provided by Melnyk and Fineout-Overholt (2005, 2011) as follows:

■ Level I: Evidence from a systematic review or meta-analysis of all relevant randomized controlled trials (RCTs), or evidence-based clinical practice guidelines based on systematic reviews of RCTs

- Level II: Evidence obtained from at least one well-designed RCT
- Level III: Evidence obtained from well-designed controlled trials without randomization
- Level IV: Evidence from well-designed, case-control and cohort studies
- Level V: Evidence from systematic reviews of descriptive and qualitative studies
- Level VI: Evidence from a single descriptive or qualitative study
- Level VII: Evidence from the opinion of authorities and/or reports of expert committees. (Melnyk & Fineout-Overholt, 2005, 2011)

These and many other tools can be used to evaluate the quality of a guideline and the evidence that informed the guideline. APNs evaluating guidelines and the evidence will need to select which tool to use. However, it is important to appreciate the differences among various tools as well as the significance of a guideline in altering clinical practice and the possibility of not achieving the preferred outcome because of challenges involved in changing clinical practice.

Comparative Effectiveness Research

Innovations in pharmaceuticals and therapeutic interventions have resulted in a tremendous amount of treatment options for clinicians, patients, and insurers. As the state of the evidence evolves, often little is known or widely understood about the relative effectiveness of these various options. Efforts to compare the effectiveness among these options for a specific condition can focus on the benefits and risks of each option, or the costs and benefits of those options. In some instances, one of the options may prove to be more effective clinically or more cost effective for a broad range of patients. However, a key issue is determining which specific type(s) of patient(s) would benefit most from a specific option.

Comparative effectiveness research (CER) is defined by the IOM as "the generation and synthesis of evidence that compares the benefits and harms of alternative methods to prevent, diagnose, treat, and monitor a clinical condition or to improve the delivery of care. The purpose of CER is to assist consumers, practitioners, purchasers, and policy makers to make informed decisions that will improve health care at both the individual and population levels" (IOM, 2009, p. 29). The core question of CER is which treatment works best, for whom, and under what circumstances. Findings from CER can provide invaluable information for clinical and coverage-related decision making. While the importance of CER increases, there continues to be both technical and policy-related questions about how CER is conducted, disseminated, and utilized.

Over the past few years, the federal government has made a substantial investment in CER. The American Recovery and Reinvestment Act of 2009 provided $1.1 billion for CER, dividing that money among the Office of the Secretary in the U.S. Department of Health and Human Services, the National Institutes of Health, and the AHRQ. Then in March of 2010, Congress passed the Affordable Care Act, which created the Patient Centered Outcomes Research Institute, a non-governmental body that will establish a nationwide agenda for the research, much of which will be funded by a tax imposed on health insurers. The purpose of this institute is to review evidence and produce new information on how diseases, disorders, and other health conditions can be treated to achieve the best clinical outcome for patients. One of the organizations providing leadership in the area of CER is the AHRQ.

Revising Existing Standards, Guidelines, and Protocols

Standards, guidelines, and protocols that were developed more than 5 years ago, and in some instances less than 5 years ago, may be out of date given more recent published research evidence. As research evolves with new information, guidelines need to be updated perhaps as often as every three years to reflect changes in empirical knowledge. Additionally, because of the availability of new research evidence varies by topic, guidelines generally become outdated in 5.8 years (Shekelle et al., 2000).

CHANGING PRACTICE

To implement evidence-based practices in many organizations, decision makers need to balance the strengths and limitations of all relevant research evidence with the practical realities of the practice environment and patient population. This includes consideration of the clinical usefulness, the limitations of the available evidence, and understanding of the differentiation that exists among the multiple, evidence-based practices for the same issue (Anderson et al., 2005). From a practical standpoint, evidence-based guidelines have to be tailored to the organization and the unique subculture(s) within.

Practitioners that want to improve the quality, safety, effectiveness, and efficiency of health care services can apply research evidence and best practices. Yet, practitioners are challenged to find, assess, interpret, and apply the current best evidence. Evidence is increasingly accessible through publications and information services such as electronic databases, systematic reviews, and health care journals. However, there are challenges to the successful application of the best information to changing practice.

To provide guidance on which factors practitioners should consider when determining whether research findings from a study should inform practice changes, the following has been proposed:

Factors related to the study in question:

1. The study should be of the highest possible quality (e.g., important and testable clinical question, prospective, large enough, randomized, blinded, controlled, minimal sources of bias).
2. The study results should be the best information available.
3. The study results should be valid and plausible.
4. The benefits of the change should outweigh the risks of implementing the change.

Factors not related to the study in question:

1. The costs of changing (or not changing) practice must be assessed.
2. The similarity of your clinical setting to that of the study.
3. The similarity of your health care system to that of the study.
4. "Expert" opinion and regulation (Cone & Lewis, 2003, p. 418).

Researchers have found that guidelines have minimal impact on changing physician behavior (Hayward, 1997; Woolf, 1993), but this could be due to a "lack of awareness, lack of familiarity, lack of agreement, lack of self-efficacy, lack of outcome expectancy, the inertia of previous practice, and external barriers" (Cabana et al., 1999, p. 1463). There may be similar issues for nurses (Creedon, 2005; Lyerla, 2008), yet several studies have indicated that nurses are more compliant with guidelines than physicians (Erasmus et al., 2010). However, one of the most significant challenges for nurses using guidelines is that much of the nursing knowledge has not been translated into evidence-based guidelines. Also, research is needed to understand the challenges faced by APNs and their compliance with guidelines to determine opportunities for improvement.

Determining Which Guidelines to Use in Practice

Before a guideline is adopted or translated into practice, clinicians and organizations should critically review the guideline. There are two approaches to evaluating guidelines for potential use in clinical practice. The Appraisal of Guidelines for Research and Evaluation (AGREE) collaboration developed an evaluation instrument with 23 criteria for appraising the process used to produce clinical practice guidelines (Exhibit 7.1). The instrument is organized using six domains: 1) scope and purpose; 2) stakeholder involvement; 3) rigor of development; 4) clarity; 5) applicability; and 6) editorial independence (AGREE, 2001). The other approach uses the Grading of Recommendations, Assessment, Development, and Evaluation (GRADE) system which grades both the evidence and strength of the recommendation, taking into account the

EXHIBIT 7.1

AGREE Instrument

SCOPE AND PURPOSE
1. The overall objective(s) of the guideline is (are) specifically described.
2. The clinical questions(s) covered by the guideline is (are) specifically described.
3. The patients to whom the guideline is meant to apply are specifically described.

STAKEHOLDER INVOLVEMENT
4. The guideline development group includes individuals from all the relevant professional groups.
5. The patients' views and preferences have been sought.
6. The target users of the guideline are clearly defined.
7. The guideline has been piloted among target users.

RIGOR OF DEVELOPMENT
8. Systematic methods were used to search for evidence.
9. The criteria for selecting the evidence are clearly described.
10. The methods used for formulating the recommendations are clearly described.
11. The health benefits, side effects, and risks have been considered in formulating the recommendations.
12. There is an explicit link between the recommendations and the supporting evidence.
13. The guideline has been externally reviewed by experts prior to its publication.
14. A procedure for updating the guideline is provided.

CLARITY AND PRESENTATION
15. The recommendations are specific and unambiguous.
16. The different options for management of the condition are clearly presented.
17. Key recommendations are easily identifiable.
18. The guideline is supported with tools for application.

APPLICABILITY
19. The potential organizational barriers in applying the recommendations have been discussed.
20. The potential cost implications of applying the recommendations have been considered.
21. The guideline presents key review criteria for monitoring and/or audit purposes.

EDITORIAL INDEPENDENCE
22. The guideline is editorially independent from the funding body.
23. Conflicts of interest of guideline development members have been recorded.

From the AGREE Collaboration. (2001). Appraisal of Guidelines for Research & Evaluation (AGREE) Instrument, 2001.

design of the research studies, the quality of the studies, and the consistency of the findings.

The purpose of the GRADE system is to guide clinicians about which studies are likely to be the most valid by taking into account more than just the quality of the research evidence. Using this system, recommendations are graded on five factors including: 1) certainty regarding the benefits, risks, and inconvenience; 2) the size of the benefit produced; 3) the importance of the benefit produced; 4) the precision of the benefit estimate; and 5) the cost. This system also grades the quality of the evidence and the strength of the recommendations according to the following factors: 1) quality of evidence for each outcome; 2) relative importance of outcomes; 3) overall quality of the evidence; 4) balance of benefits and harms; 5) balance of net benefits and costs; 6) strength of the recommendation; and 7) implementation and evaluation (Atkins et al., 2004).

Getting Research Into Practice

After the research and evidence and/or guidelines have been identified and evaluated for application to practice, getting research-based evidence into practice requires applying evidence-based recommendations at the right time, in the right place, and in the right way. Yet, there are most likely several barriers to implementation, from the organizational level to the actual process of care. First, senior staff and management must be committed to change and enable that change through resource allocation and policies. Second, leaders and clinicians must be invested in making the necessary changes to implement evidence into practice. Third, it is often necessary to make changes in how care is organized and how it is delivered, which may not be acceptable to some clinicians. Fourth, clinicians will need skill development and training to successfully utilize the evidence in practice. Fifth, it is important to ensure that clinicians have the tools they need to successfully use the evidence in practice, such as computerized decision support tools. Finally, it is important to build alliances with key partners and share ownership in ensuring the success of implementation and continued utilization of the evidence in practice. If any of these organizational level factors are not in place and functioning well, efforts to implement the evidence/guideline into practice may be thwarted or may be successful initially then fail over time.

While the goal of evidence-based guidelines is to standardize care across settings and practitioners, there are aspects that need to be tailored to the patient and the patient's circumstances. Because the delivery of health care involves complex decisions, simply implementing evidence/guidelines will not necessarily meet individual patient needs (Clancy & Cronin, 2005). In practice, practitioners need to integrate the best evidence, clinical expertise, patient preferences, and patient values in making decisions (Sackett et al., 2000).

Given the importance of patient- and family-centered care, practitioners need to consider involving patients in the decision-making process. Practitioners must be able to define each patient's unique circumstances, determine what is wrong with the patient, and assess how the condition is affecting the patient. Once the possible interventions and treatments are discussed with the patient, the patient may be opposed to the recommended interventions and care management plan. Using a patient-centered care approach injects the patient's preferences, values, and rights into the process of deciding on which interventions to use and the appropriate management. While this is appropriate and encouraged by policy makers and decision makers, guidelines, standards, and protocols are generally written in such a way that assumes patient consent to the evidence. As such, it is important to integrate research evidence into clinical decision making and to customize it to the patient's clinical circumstances and wishes, thereby deriving a meaningful decision about interventions and care management.

Evaluating Your Practice Outcomes

As important as using evidence in practice is, it is also important to understand the impact of both non-evidence-based practices and evidence-based practices on care processes and outcomes. Many organizations and practitioners continue to make the mistake of implementing evidence-based or evidence-informed changes in care processes, but fail to measure the impact on care processes as well as patient and organizational outcomes. This is a significant failure because there is always a cost associated with changes in care processes and decision making, and assuming that implementing evidence/guidelines will result in better outcomes cannot be proven unless appropriately measured and assessed. At a basic level, outcomes should be assessed before and after a change is made.

SUMMARY

Patient and organizational outcomes can be improved and a consistency in care across settings and practitioners achieved by applying evidence and clinical standards, guidelines, and protocols to practice. There are many influences on what evidence is available and how it may be used in practice. Practitioners and patients need to be actively involved in using the best evidence to inform decision making and improve outcomes.

REFERENCES

Academy Health. (2005). *Placement, coordination, and funding of health services research within the federal government.* Washington, DC: Academy Health Report.

Agency for Healthcare Research and Quality. (2010, October). *Evidence-based practice centers overview.* Rockville, MD: Agency for healthcare research and quality. Retrieved from http://www.ahrq.gov/clinic/epc

AGREE Collaboration. (2001). *Appraisal of guidelines for research & evaluation (AGREE) instrument.* Retrieved from http://www.agreecollaboration.org/pdf/agreeinstrumentfinal.pdf

American Nurses Association. *Standards.* Retrieved from www.nursingworld.org/MainMenuCategories/ThePracticeofProfessionalNursing/NursingStandards.aspx.

American Nurses Association. (2004). *Nursing: Scope & standards of practice.* Washington, DC: Author.

American Nurses Association. (2010). *Nursing: Scope & standards of practice* (2nd ed.). Washington, DC: Author.

Anderson, L. M., Brownson, R. C., Fullilove, M. T., Teutsch, S. M., Novick, L. F., Fielding, J., & Land, G. H. (2005). Evidence-based public health policy and practice: Promises and limits. *American Journal of Preventive Medicine, 28*(5S), 226–230.

Atkins, D., Eccles, M., Flottorp, S., Guyatt, G. H., Henry, D., Hill, S., … Williams, J. W., Jr.; GRADE Working Group. (2004). Systems for grading the quality of evidence and the strength of recommendations I: Critical appraisal of existing approaches. The Grade Working Group. *BMC Health Services Research, 4*, 38. Retrieved from http://www.biomedcentral.com/1472-6963/4/38

Baker, R. (2001). Is it time to review the idea of compliance with guidelines? *British Journal of General Practice, 51*, 7.

Balas, E. A., & Boren, S. A. (2002). *Managing clinical knowledge for health care improvement. Yearbook of medical informatics.* Powerpoint presentation. Retrieved from www.socialresearchmethods.net.

Bates, D. W., Kuperman, G. J., Wang, S., Gandhi, T., Kittler, A., Volk, L., … Middleton, B. (2003). Ten commandments for effective clinical decision support: Making the practice of evidence-based medicine a reality. *Journal of the American Medical Informatics Association, 10*(6), 523–530.

Cabana, M. D., Rand, C. S., Powe, N. R., Wu, A. W., Wilson, M. H., Abboud, P. A., & Rubin, H. R. (1999). Why don't physicians follow clinical practice guidelines? A framework for improvement. *Journal of the American Medical Association, 282*(15), 1458–1467.

Clancy, C., & Cronin, K. (2005). Evidence-based decision making: Global evidence, local decisions. *Health Affairs, 24*(1), 151–162.

Closs, S. J., & Cheater, F. M. (1999). Evidence for nursing practice: A clarification of the issues. *Journal of Advanced Nursing, 30*(1), 10–17.

College of Registered Nurses of Nova Scotia. (2004). *Standards for nursing practice.* Retrieved from http://www.crnns.ca/documents/standards2004.pdf

Cone, D. C., & Lewis, R. J. (2003). Should this study change my practice? *Academic Emergency Medicine, 10*(5), 417–422.

Creedon S. A. (2005). Healthcare workers' hand decontamination practices: Compliance with recommended guidelines. *Journal of Advanced Nursing, 51*(3), 208–216.

Eccles M. P., & Grimshaw J. M. (2004). Selecting, presenting and delivering clinical guidelines: Are there any "magic bullets"? *Medical Journal of Australia, 180* (Suppl. 6), S52–S54.

Emanuel, L. L. (1997). Professional standards in health care: Calling all parties to account. *Health Affairs, 16*(1), 52–54.

Erasmus, V., Daha, T. J., Brug, H., Richardus, J. H., Behrendt, M. D., Vos, M. C., & van Beeck, E. F. (2010). Systematic review of studies on compliance with hand hygiene guidelines in hospital care. *Infection Control Hospital Epidemiology, 31*(3), 283–294.

Feder, G., Eccles, M., Grol, R., Griffiths, C., & Grimshaw, J. (1999). Using clinical guidelines. *British Medical Journal, 318*(7185), 728–730.

Field, M. J., & Lohr, K. N. (Eds.), (1990). *Clinical practice guidelines: Directions for a new program. Institute of medicine, Committee to advise the public health services on clinical practice guidelines.* Washington, DC: National Academy Press.

Guyatt, G., Vist, G., Falck-Ytter, Y., Kunz, R., Magrini, N., Schünemann, H., & Elena, R. (2006). An emerging consensus on grading recommendations. *ACP Journal Club,* A8–A9.

Hayward, R. S. A. (1997). Clinical practice guidelines on trial. *CMAJ, 156,* 1725–1727.

Health Information and Management Systems Society. (2010). *Dictionary of health-care information technology terms, acronyms and organizations* (2nd ed.). Chicago, IL: Author.

Institute of Medicine. (2001). *Crossing the quality chasm.* Washington, DC: National Academy Press.

Institute of Medicine. (2004a). *Keeping patients safe: Transforming the work environment of nurses.* Washington, DC: National Academy Press.

Institute of Medicine. (2004b). *Patient safety: Achieving a new standard for care.* Washington, DC: National Academy Press.

Institute of Medicine. (2008). *Knowing what works in health care: A roadmap for the nation.* Washington, DC: National Academy Press.

Institute of Medicine. (2009). *Initial national priorities for comparative effectiveness research.* Washington, DC: National Academy Press.

Institute of Medicine. (2011a). *Clinical practice guidelines we can trust.* Washington, DC: National Academy Press.

Institute of Medicine. (2011b). *What works in health care: Standards for systematic reviews.* Washington, DC: National Academy Press.

Joint Commission. (2008). *About the joint commission.* Retrieved from http://www.jointcommission.org/about_us/about_the_joint_commission_main.aspx

Joint Commission. (2011a). *National patient safety goals.* Retrieved from http://www.jointcommission.org/standards_information/npsgs.aspx

Joint Commission. (2011b). *Specifications manual for national hospital inpatient quality measures.* Retrieved from http://www.jointcommission.org/specifications_manual_for_national_hospital_inpatient_quality_measures

Kohn, L. T., Corrigan, J. M., & Donaldson, M. S. (Eds.), (2000). *To err is human: Building a safer health system. A report of the committee on quality of health care in America, institute of medicine.* Washington, DC: National Academy Press.

Lomas, J., Sisk, J. E., & Stocking, B. (1993). From evidence to practice in the United States, the United Kingdom, and Canada. *Milbank Quarterly, 71*(3), 405–410.

Lyerla, F. (2008). Design and implementation of a nursing clinical decision support system to promote guideline adherence. *Computer Informatics Nursing, 26*(4), 227–233.

McGlynn, E., Asch, S., Adams, J., Keesey, J., Hicks, J., Decristofaro, A., & Kerr, E. (2003). The quality of health care delivered to adults in the United States. *New England Journal of Medicine, 348*(26), 2635–2645.

Melnyk, B. M., & Fineout-Overholt, E. (2005). *Evidence-based practice in nursing & healthcare. A guide to best practice.* Philadelphia, PA: Lippincott Williams & Wilkins.

Melnyk, B. M., & Fineout-Overholt, E. (2011). *Evidence-based practice in nursing & healthcare* (2nd ed.). Philadelphia, PA: Lippincott Williams & Wilkins.

Moffett, P., & Moore, G. (2011). The standard of care: Legal history and definitions. *Western Journal of Emergency Medicine, 12*(1), 109–112.

Moses, H., III, Dorsey, E. R., Matheson, D. H., & Their, S. O. (2005). Financial anatomy of biomedical research. *Journal of the American Medical Association, 294*(11), 1333–1242.

Newhouse, R. P., Dearholt, S., Poe, S., Pugh, L. C., & White, K. M. (2007). Organizational change strategies for evidence-based practice. *Journal of Nursing Administration, 37*(12), 552–557.

Robert Wood Johnson Foundation. (2004). *A guide to evaluation of primers.* Retrieved from http://www.rwjf.org/pr/product.jsp?id=18657

Sackett, D., Strauss, S., & Richardson, W., Rosenberg, W. S., & Haynes, R. B. (2000). *Evidence based medicine: How to practice and teach EBM.* New York: Churchill Livingstone.

Shekelle, P., Woolf, S. K., & Eccles, M., (2000). Developing guidelines. In M. Eccles & J. Grimshaw (Eds.), *Clinical practice guidelines: From conception to use.* Oxford, UK: Radclliffe Medical Press.

Shekelle, P. G., Woolf, S. H., Eccles, M., & Grimshaw, J. (1999). Developing guidelines. *British Medical Journal, 318,* 593–596.

Shekelle, P. G., Ortiz, E., Rhodes, S., Morton, S. C., Eccles, M. P., Grimshaw. J. M., & Woolf, S. H. (2001). Validity of the agency for healthcare research and quality clinical practice guidelines: How quickly do guidelines become outdated? *Journal of the American Medical Association, 286*(12), 1461–1467.

Stillwell, S. B., Fineout-Overhold, E., Melynk, B. M., & Williamson, K. M. (2010). Evidence-based practice, step by step: Asking the clinical question: A key step in evidence-based practice. *American Journal of Nursing, 110*(3), 58–61.

Timmermans, S., & Berg, M. (2003). *The gold standard: The challenge of evidence-based medicine and standardization in health care.* Philadelphia, PA: Temple University Press.

U.S. Preventive Services Task Force Grade Definitions. (2008, May). Retrieved from http://www.uspreventiveservicestaskforce.org/uspstf/grades.htm

U.S. Preventive Services Task Force Ratings: Grade Definitions. Guide to clinical preventive services, third edition: Periodic updates, 2000-2003. Retrieved from http://www.uspreventiveservicestaskforce.org/3rduspstf/ratings.htm

Woolf, S. H. (1993). Practice guidelines: A new reality in medicine, III: Impact on patient care. *Archives of Internal Medicine, 153,* 2646–2655.

Woolf, S. H., Grol, R., Hutchinson, A., Eccles, M., & Grimshaw, J. (1999). Clinical guidelines: Potential benefits, limitations, and harms of clinical guidelines. *British Medical Journal, 318*(7182), 527–530.

EIGHT

Evaluating Populations and Population Health

Deanna E. Grimes and Nancy F. Weller

"The health of the people is really the foundation upon which all their happiness and all their powers as a state depend."

Benjamin Disraeli

INTRODUCTION

There was a time when the health of populations was considered to be the purview of public health agencies and public/community health workers, specifically nurses. Then, health care organizations and providers framed their responsibilities in terms of the populations served, such as workers in an industry, school children, residents of a long-term care facility or enrollees in a managed care organization. Today, APNs recognize an expansion of their role from simply caring for individual patients in a clinic/hospital/nursing home, to caring for a panel of patients seen regularly in those settings. APNs also recognize that their patients have health problems similar to those of the populations from which they come. In this time of promoting efficiency in health care, it is not always efficient to treat population health problems that could be prevented. APNs increasingly find themselves working to change health and health care for the populations served.

The American Association of Colleges of Nursing (AACN) recognized the importance of focusing on the health of populations in their document *The Essentials of Doctoral Education for Advanced Nursing Practice*. The focus of Essential VII is clinical prevention and population health for improving the nation's health (AACN, 2006). The AACN (2006, p. 16) outlined the expectations of the doctoral nursing graduate as follows:

1. Analyze epidemiological, biostatistical, environmental, and other appropriate scientific data related to individual, aggregate, and population health.
2. Synthesize concepts, including psychosocial dimensions and cultural diversity, related to clinical prevention and population health in developing, implementing, and evaluating interventions to address health promotion/disease prevention efforts, improve health status/ access patterns, and/or address gaps in care of individuals, aggregates, or populations.
3. Evaluate care delivery models and/or strategies using concepts related to community, environmental and occupational health, and cultural and socioeconomic dimensions of health.

How can an APN apply the requirements of Essential VII into practice? A case study on TB is presented in the following to highlight population-focused concepts/methods that may serve as a guide for the APN in the application of Essential VII requirements to his/her practice.

APNs are frequently faced with implementing patient- or population-focused guidelines, such as the updated TB guidelines, in a variety of

CASE STUDY

In 2005, the Centers for Disease Control and Prevention (CDC) published an update to their guidelines for preventing the transmission of *Mycobacterium tuberculosis* in health care settings (CDC, 2005). These new guidelines emphasized that health care organizations assess and categorize the risk for transmission of TB in their settings prior to implementing the guidelines. The guidelines cover valuable information directed to clinic/hospital administrators, clinicians, and TB control personnel on such topics as:

a. Health care workers who should be included in a TB surveillance program
b. Pathogenesis, epidemiology, and transmission of *M. tuberculosis*
c. Persons at highest risk for exposure to and infection with *M. tuberculosis*
d. Persons who are at high risk for progression to TB disease
e. Characteristics of a patient with TB disease that increases the risk for infectiousness
f. Environmental factors that increase the probability of transmission
g. Risk for health care-associated transmission of *M. tuberculosis*
h. TB risk assessment in populations, and so on.

different settings. What are the principles illustrated in this case that can be used by APNs in any setting? The following questions will be the focus of the remainder of this chapter: 1) What is a population and what is the definition of population health? 2) What is meant by the terms risk, risk factors, and populations at risk? 3) What are the determinants of health that may contribute to risk? 4) How does one assess the distribution of a disease, such as TB, in a population? 5) How does one assess risk factors and populations at risk for TB? 6) What models may be used to analyze a health problem and disease in a population? 7) How does one evaluate the impact of an intervention on the health problem?

POPULATIONS AND POPULATION HEALTH

Population, as a general term, refers to a group of people who have a common characteristic, such as age, geography, political boundaries, race/ethnicity, religion, environmental exposures, occupation, education, sexual preference, and so on. According to the AACN, population health includes "aggregate, community, environmental/occupational, and cultural/socioeconomic dimensions of health. Aggregates are groups of individuals defined by a shared characteristic such as gender, diagnosis, or age" (AACN, 2006, p. 15).

In the field of health and health care, populations are identified by their health status or medical condition, such as persons with a disability or with a TB infection or active TB disease. They are also identified by their risk for certain conditions: smokers are at risk for lung cancer and persons with HIV infection are at risk for active TB disease. For example, the 2005 CDC guidelines on TB referred to four different populations at risk for TB: 1) the geographic community (local, regional, state, national) from which TB cases derived; 2) population groups that are at greatest risk for obtaining or transmitting TB, such as the homeless; 3) patients in a variety of health care settings, including clinics and nursing homes; and 4) the many categories of health care workers exposed to TB at their places of employment.

How do you, as an APN, define the population you serve? How would you define population health relative to your population? With respect to the tuberculosis case study, who is the population served by the nursing administrator of a hospital? Who is the population served by an APN in an outpatient clinic? Who is the population served by the triage nurse in the emergency department?

RISK, RISK FACTORS, POPULATIONS AT RISK

Risk and assessment of risk are major foci of the CDC guidelines on TB. The guidelines identified risk associated with the transmission of TB, risk factors in certain groups that increase the risk of transmitting TB, populations at risk for acquiring TB infection, and populations at risk for acquiring TB disease.

Risk is simply the probability that something will occur. With respect to health, risk is the increased probability that a disease, injury, disability, or death will occur to an individual or a population. The term is generally applied to the probability that something specific will occur, such as the risk of infection with *M. tuberculosis*. *Risk factors* are those characteristics of an individual and/ or a population that increase their risk for disease, illness, disability, or death. Living in proximity to a person with active TB is a risk factor for acquiring *M. tuberculosis*. The term *populations at risk* refers to all those persons who have a similar type of risk, such as health care workers with continuing exposure to patients with active TB infection. Individuals who are immune compromised are a population at risk for TB infection that can progress to active TB disease.

DETERMINANTS OF HEALTH

Apart from risk and risk factors, why are some people healthy and others not? What are the conditions that contribute to disparities in health among individuals and populations? These conditions are commonly called the *determinants of health*. Determinants of health are the array of personal, social, economic and environmental factors that impact the health status of populations. These determinants have been defined more formally as the "combined effects of individual and community physical and social environments and the policies and interventions used to promote health, prevent disease, and ensure access to quality health care" (U.S. Department of Health and Human Services [USDHHS], 2002, p. 7). A model for the determinants of health can be seen in Figure 8.1.

Since the term *determinants of health* was coined, the number and types or categories of determinants have varied. Originally there were four general determinants (human biology, health system, environment, and lifestyle) included in the Lalonde Report (Glouberman & Miller, 2003). The determinants of health depicted in the *Healthy People 2010* (Figure 8.1) and the *Healthy People 2020* documents include biology and genetics, social environment, physical environment, health services or access to quality health care, policies and interventions, and individual behaviors or lifestyle (USDHHS, 2001, 2009). These six categories of determinants are described in the following.

Social Environment

Social factors include relationships with family and friends, workplace colleagues, neighbors, and other community members. Social environment may also include access to resources in the community (public safety, parks and recreational facilities), social institutions (law enforcement, school systems, governmental and social service agencies), and cultural features and practices.

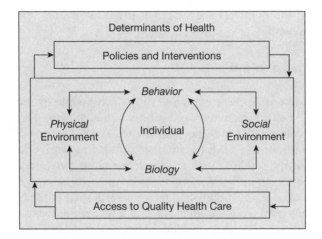

FIGURE 8.1
The Healthy People Model for Determinant of Health.
From the U.S. Department of Health and Human Services
(n.d.). Healthy People 2010: A systematic approach. Retrieved
from http://www.healthypeople.gov/2010/Document/html/
uih/uih_2.htm#deter

Social factors may directly or indirectly affect health, as their effects may accumulate across time and the lifespans of individuals, and across generations of individuals and families. The social environment may lead to undesirable cycles between these social factors and health. Although genes and access to good health care are important overall, social factors may play a larger role than either genetics or health services because they interact with both. Fortunately, many of these social factors may be influenced by policies and programs designed and targeted to remediate their harmful effects. Many models of the social determinants of health, both early and especially later versions of these expanding models, include the following social factors: early life experience, education, income, housing, community, race/ethnicity, occupation/work, and the economy (USDHHS, 2009).

With respect to the case study on TB, the social environment may impact the spread of disease. Economic conditions may force some persons to live in crowded conditions increasing the risk of transmission of the pathogen. Immigrant families, especially those within 5 years of arrival from geographic areas with a high incidence of TB disease, may be infected without awareness. They may live together in one apartment or in close proximity in congested urban neighborhoods and may be at greater risk for transmission of TB. Those isolated from resources because of language barriers may not have access to health care, particularly screening for TB infection. Residents and employees of congregate settings that are high risk (e.g., correctional facilities, long-term care facilities, and homeless shelters) may also be at greater risk due to their social environment.

Physical Environment

Physical conditions in the environment in which people live, recreate, and work impact health, functioning, and quality of life. Examples of the physical determinants of health include: housing, homes, and neighborhoods; exposure to toxins and physical hazards (accumulated trash and debris); physical barriers to those with disabilities (lack of wheelchair ramps); natural environment (plants, weather, air quality); man-made environment (buildings); occupational settings; educational institutions; and recreational areas (USDHHS, 2009). Poor quality housing may expose residents to undesirable conditions and contribute to poorer health. Inferior and substandard housing may lead to infectious diseases, injuries, exposure to lead, which is dangerous to children under the age of 6, and other household toxins. In the case of TB, close contacts may expose others to TB disease. Close contacts are persons who share the same air space in a household or other enclosed environment for a prolonged period (days or weeks, not minutes or hours) with a person with pulmonary TB disease.

Policies and Interventions

Governmental policies at the local, state, and federal levels may profoundly affect individual and population health. Individual- and population-level behavior change may occur with changes in government regulations. Cuts in programs, such as Medicaid, to dependent and low-income families due to changes in political structure at the state and federal level may greatly alter the resources of struggling, working-class families. In the case of TB, changing the restrictions on immigration between and among nations with a high incidence of TB may alter the numbers of high-risk TB cases coming into the United States. Most state public health agencies currently cover the cost of treatment with anti-TB drugs and for directly observed therapy (DOT) programs. Changes in how treatment is financed could dramatically alter the health outcomes for those with TB and those with whom they come in contact.

Health Services or Access to Quality Health Care

Lack of or limited access to quality health services may seriously erode population health. The failure to maintain health insurance policies due to poverty and/or unemployment or underemployment, for example, may lessen participation in preventive health care and delay needed medical treatment. In addition to those already mentioned, barriers to health services include high cost of care, limited language access, and immigration status. These barriers lead to unmet health needs, delays in receiving needed care, lack of preventive care, and unnecessary hospitalizations. Lack of access to quality health care serves to increase health disparities among racial/ethnic and socioeconomic groups, profoundly affecting the health of certain components of the population (USDHHS, 2009). Populations who are medically underserved and who have low income may be at greater risk for exposure to and infection with TB; the infant, school-age and adolescent children, of these medically underserved adults, especially those with compromised immune function such as HIV, may be at high risk for exposure and acquisition of disease.

Individual Behaviors or Lifestyle

Individual behaviors and lifestyle choices may also impact health outcomes. These factors include an individual's responses to internal stimuli and external conditions and often interact with an individual's biology. Lifestyle factors include risk behaviors, such as alcohol, tobacco, and other kinds of substance abuse; unprotected sexual behaviors; sedentary lifestyle and lack of regular physical activity; poor diet; and poor safety practices, such as seat belt and child restraint use in motor vehicles. Persons who use tobacco, alcohol, or illegal drugs, including injection drugs and crack cocaine, might also be at increased risk for infection and TB disease. Many population health interventions target such individual behaviors, reducing the rates of chronic disease and injury acquired from risky behaviors.

Biology and Genetics

Biological factors include the effects of an individual's genetic makeup, family history, and physical and mental health problems acquired over the course of the individual's lifetime. Genetic factors may affect certain population groups more than others. Older individuals are more likely to acquire cancers due to the physical effects of aging on cells. Examples of genetic and biological determinants of health include: age, gender, immune status, certain inherited conditions (sickle cell anemia, hemophilia, and cystic fibrosis); the *BRCA1* or *BRCA2* gene, which increases the risk of breast and ovarian cancer; and a family history of certain forms of heart disease (USDHHS, 2009). Those who are immune compromised in any manner, including those with HIV infection, have an increased risk for progression from latent TB infection to TB disease.

ASSESSING THE DISTRIBUTION OF DISEASE IN A POPULATION

How would one apply the previous discussion of risk and determinants of health in order to implement the 2005 TB prevention guidelines? The guidelines (CDC, 2005, Appendix B) ask the following: 1) What is the incidence of TB in your community (county or region served by the health care setting), and how does it compare with the state and national average? 2) What is the incidence of TB in your facility and specific settings, and how do those rates compare? 3) Are patients with suspected or confirmed TB disease encountered in your setting (inpatient and outpatient)? If yes, how many are treated in your health care setting in 1 year? 4) Currently, does your health care setting have a cluster of persons with confirmed TB disease that might be a result of ongoing transmission of *M. tuberculosis*?

A review of basic concepts and methods pertaining to these measures of morbidity may be helpful here. *Distribution of disease* refers to the occurrence of a disease, injury, disability, or death according to the extent of the problem in the population during a time period. The common questions are: What is the disease or other health problem? How much is occurring? To whom? And when? If one is counting new events in nursing staff, such as new TB infection cases diagnosed by positive conversions of the TB skin test, the new infections are called *incidence*. Newly diagnosed active TB disease during a time period also is incidence. A count of all of the staff demonstrating a positive TB skin test at one time, regardless of when they were infected, is called *prevalence*. All patients treated for active TB disease and attending a TB clinic over a time period are referred to as prevalent cases.

It is also important to relate cases, whether new or existing, to the population from which they were counted. This process involves relating the cases (the numerator) to the whole (the denominator) to calculate a proportion, percentage, or rate. *Rates* are the basic measures of disease, injury, disability, or death in a defined population over a specified period of time. Rates allow comparisons between populations, between geographic areas, and over periods of time. *Incidence rates* are calculated by the number of events occurring in a population during a specific time period, divided by the number of persons in the population at risk for those events, and multiplied by a base number (100, 1000, 10,000, or 100,000) that will result in a whole number answer. For example, one might calculate the incidence rate of TB during 2011 in a county as:

$$\frac{\text{Number of new cases of TB in 2011}}{\text{Number of residents in the country in 2011}} \times 100,000 = \frac{\text{TB incidence per}}{\text{100,000 population}}$$

Prevalence rates are calculated by the number of existing events in a population during a time period or at one time, divided by the number of persons in the population at risk for those events, multiplied by a base number (100, 1000, 10,000, or 100,000) that will result in a whole number.

$$\frac{\text{Number of persons with TB hospitalized today}}{\text{Total number of patients in the hospital today}} \times 100 = \frac{\text{\% of hospitalized}}{\text{patients with TB}}$$
(Subtract the TB cases from this number)

The 2005 CDC guidelines for TB also specify that the incidence rates of new TB cases should be compared with a state or national distribution of the disease. The state or national distribution of TB is sometimes called a *standard* population, that is, one that encompasses the population being studied. The process of comparison is similar to comparing one's weight with a standard weight chart for one's height and age. State or national TB incidence rates serve as a *standard* for comparing the local or regional rates. Therefore, assessment of the distribution of TB could include comparison of incidence rates of TB in the local population during the past year with those of the state or nation during the same time period, as well as incidence over time, incidence in certain high risk groups, and incidence in the health care facility or clinic.

Additionally, it is important to assess the characteristics of the populations who have TB disease and who have TB infection. What are their demographic characteristics such as ages, genders, race or ethnicity? Where do they live (urban, rural, or suburban areas)? What is the geography and climate of their locale? What are their living conditions (single-family dwellings, multiple-family households, congregate living facilities)? What do members of the population do for a living and where do they work? Do they have co-morbidities, such as cancers or HIV, that may exacerbate their infection with TB?

Because TB disease is a reportable condition, data on the numbers and rates of TB disease in the local, regional, and state geographic areas are available from local and state health departments and from the CDC. The presence of TB disease in health care facilities may be monitored by laboratory data and patient records. TB infection, as determined by skin testing, is not reportable to local health departments.

ASSESSING RISK FACTORS AND POPULATIONS AT RISK

Understanding the mechanisms whereby a disease or health problem exists in a population provides a roadmap for assessing risk factors for the condition in the population. With respect to an infectious disease, an examination of such factors as the nature and virulence of the pathogen, mode of transmission, natural history of the disease, susceptibility of the potential host, and environmental factors that may increase the probability of transmission, are important to understand in terms of disease control and prevention.

As discussed earlier in this chapter, risk and assessment of risk are major foci of the CDC guidelines. APNs are frequently responsible for the care of populations afflicted by infectious disease, for example, H1N1 influenza, which is also spread by droplet transmission. The principles inherent in these guidelines may be used by the APN in caring for patient populations, by the hospital/clinic administrator responsible for the health of the staff, and by ancillary personnel who contact ill patients.

The guidelines identified risk associated with transmission of TB, risk factors in certain groups that increase the risk of transmitting TB, populations at risk for acquiring TB infection, and populations at risk for acquiring TB disease. These are discussed in the following.

Risk Associated With Transmission of *M. tuberculosis*

M. tuberculosis is carried in airborne particles (droplet nuclei) released when persons with pulmonary or laryngeal TB disease cough, sneeze or shout. The particles are small enough that air currents may keep them airborne for prolonged periods, allowing the droplets to travel. *M. tuberculosis* is generally not transmitted by contact with surfaces that might be covered with TB particles.

Risk Factors That Increase the Risk of Transmitting TB

The more airborne particles released when a person coughs the more the risk of transmission. According to the CDC (2005), the following conditions in a person with TB increase their infectiousness: 1) cough; 2) cavitation on chest radiograph; 3) positive acid-fast bacilli sputum smear result; 4) respiratory tract disease with involvement of the larynx; 5) respiratory tract disease with involvement of the lung or pleura; 6) failure to cover the mouth and nose when coughing; 7) incorrect, lack of, or short duration of anti-tuberculosis treatment; and 8) undergoing cough-inducing or aerosol-generating procedures.

Populations at Risk for Acquiring TB Infection

Characteristics of persons exposed to *M. tuberculosis* that may increase their risk for infection are broad and sometimes ill defined. Close contact, that is, sharing the same air space for a prolonged period of time with a person with pulmonary TB disease is the major risk factor for infection. The risk of contacting someone with TB disease increases when TB is highly prevalent in the surrounding environment or in one's living quarters. So, living or working in close contact with infected persons increases the risk of acquiring the infections. The guidelines list the following as populations at risk: 1) foreign-born persons who have arrived in the United States within 5 years of moving from an area with a high incidence of TB; 2) residents and employees of congregate settings, such as homeless shelters and correctional facilities; 3) health care workers in general; 4) health care workers with unprotected exposure to a patient with TB disease; 5) low income and medically underserved populations; and 6) infants, children, and adolescents exposed to adults in high-risk categories.

The new guidelines have expanded the list of health care workers (HCW) who regularly should undergo screening for TB infection to 42. HCWs refer to all paid and unpaid persons working in health care settings who have the potential for exposure to *M. tuberculosis* through air space shared with persons with infectious TB disease. All HCWs who have duties that involve face-to-face contact with patients with suspected or confirmed TB disease (including transport staff) should be included for screening. Additionally, any employee should be screened who: 1) enters patient rooms or treatment rooms whether or not a patient is present; 2) participates in aerosol-generating or aerosol-producing procedures; 3) participates in suspected or confirmed *M. tuberculosis* specimen processing; or 4) installs, maintains, or replaces environmental controls in areas in which persons with TB disease are encountered (CDC, 2005).

Populations at Risk for Acquiring TB Disease

Not every person infected with *M. tuberculosis* will progress to have active TB disease. A compromised or undeveloped immune system seems to contribute to the progression of infection to active disease. The highest risk is for persons with HIV infection. Other groups include infants and children less than 4 years, persons with chronic and/or compromising immune conditions (silicosis; diabetes mellitus; chronic renal failure; leukemia; lymphoma; carcinoma of the head, neck or lung; prolonged corticosteroid use; other immune-suppressive treatments; organ transplant; end-stage renal disease; and intestinal bypass surgery). Additionally, persons with a history of untreated or inadequately treated TB disease and substance abusers are populations at risk for progressing to TB disease (CDC, 2005).

APNs frequently encounter infectious diseases in their practices and patient populations. Inadequate infection control practices in the health care facility increases the risk for nosocomial (health care-acquired) infections, which constitute a major population health hazard to patients, their families, and to health care professionals. The authors encourage APNs to access the CDC Guidelines for Preventing the Transmission of *Mycobacterium tuberculosis* in Health-Care Settings for more information on recognizing the risks and preventing transmission of TB (CDC, 2005).

ANALYZING A HEALTH PROBLEM IN A POPULATION

A population of patients, a geographic population, or a well population with similar characteristics (such as pregnant women or school children) may experience multiple health problems. Some are overt health status problems, such as diabetes, asthma, or TB. Others are risk factors for future health problems, such as smoking, poverty, or environmental hazards. Still others may be categorized as a lack of resources, which is the case for populations who are uninsured, homeless, or live in areas remote from health care facilities. And, some health problems do not fit into a neat category but still are expressed by patients and populations as a need—a need for help with an elderly parent, a need to have someone with whom to talk, or a need to have a place to go during a hurricane.

In order to analyze a problem, such as a high incidence of new TB infections, for possible intervention, one begins with a measure of the extent of a problem in a specific group or population, during a specific time period. Such would be the case if an APN assesses that *30% of the hospital's housekeeping staff converted to a positive TB skin test during the past year*. Although health status problems, particularly those that lead to death or are reportable infectious diseases, are the easiest to quantify in a population, it also is possible to have measures of the extent of risk factors and lack of resources. For example, an APN may have observed that *80% of the hospital's housekeeping staff do not wear respiratory protection when working in the rooms of patients in respiratory isolation.*

To plan to intervene in a problem in a population, it helps to know what is causing the problem in the population. The next step, therefore, in analyzing a health problem is to organize the evidence on determinants of the problem in the population. Some of that evidence is available from first-hand experience with the population; other evidence is available from published research and guidelines.

The authors of this chapter have used the Problem Analysis Model (Figure 8.2) to analyze complex problems in a population. The model is an adaptation of a health problem analysis worksheet that was published by the CDC, Public Health Practice Program Office in 1991 (Turnock, 2009, p. 74). The arrows at the bottom of the model represent a time line. The CDC defined a *determinant* as a "Scientifically established factor that relates directly to the level of the health problem. A health problem may have any number of determinants identified for it." For example, inhalation of *M. tuberculosis* in aerosolized mucous droplets is a determinant of infection with *M. tuberculosis.*

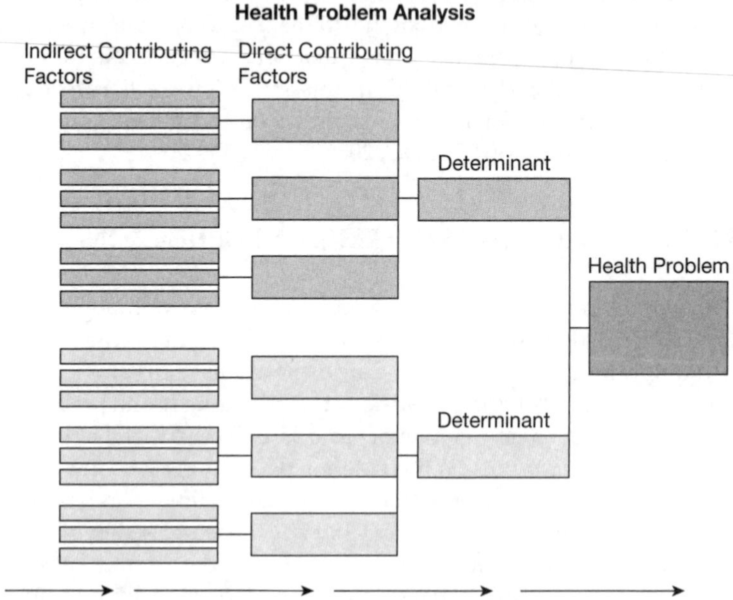

Health Problem Analysis

FIGURE 8.2
Problem Analysis Model.
Adapted from the Health Problem Analysis Worksheet,
Centers for Disease Control and Prevention, Public Health
Practice Program Office, 1991.

A *direct contributing factor* is a "Scientifically established factor that directly affects the level of the determinant." For example, near proximity to a person with active pulmonary tuberculosis is a direct contributing factor. An *indirect contributing factor* is a "Community-specific factor that affects the level of a direct contributing factor. There may be many indirect factors contributing to a direct factor and indirect factors may vary considerably from one community to another" (CDC cited by Turnock, 2009, p. 75). An example is crowded living conditions or a crowded waiting room may be an indirect contributing factor that increases the risk for exposure to the *Mycobacterium*. Figure 8.3 provides an analysis of a specific problem: 30% increase in new TB infections (diagnosed by new skin test conversions) in health care workers in one hospital.

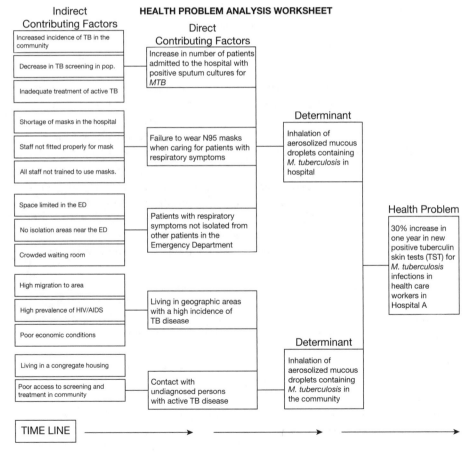

FIGURE 8.3
Example of an analysis of TB infections in hospital staff.

Note that it is easier if to start the analysis with the problem and to work backward in time and from right to left across the figure. Note, too, that the direct and indirect contributing factors provide places to intervene early to prevent the problem.

EVALUATING POPULATION HEALTH OUTCOMES

Assessing and analyzing health problems in a population are not easy tasks. They are undertaken, however, to bring about change in the problem and, ultimately, to intervene to improve the health status of the population and the individuals in the population. Multiple manuals, books, and web-based resources are available to assist organizations and health care providers to plan and implement new programs to improve the health status of the populations they serve (Exhibit 8.1). Figure 8.4 provides an overview of the process and emphasizes the ongoing and circular nature of the assessment, planning, implementation, and evaluation processes. The CDC Guidelines provide ample examples of programs and interventions to prevent transmission of *M. tuberculosis* in health care facilities.

Evaluating outcomes from a population-focused intervention is not difficult if the problem has been adequately assessed and analyzed. Evaluation officially begins when one assesses a problem according to its extent and distribution in the population. Knowing the answers to the following questions will provide guidance for the change that is desired.

- What is the extent of the problem and how is it distributed in the population?
- How does the extent compare to the extent and distribution of the problem in a standard population?
- Is the problem increasing or decreasing with time?
- Who has the problem and what are their demographic characteristics?

If one determines that the problem is greater than expected in some segments of the population, appropriate interventions then may be targeted to that population. The goal of the program would be a decrease in the extent of the problem in that population during the expected time period. Evaluation becomes straightforward: Was the stated goal achieved?

Of course, nothing ever is as easy as one would like. Let's look at the analysis of the problem of increasing TB infections in health care workers in Hospital A as seen in Figure 8.3. The authors of this chapter defined this problem as a 30% increase during the past year in new positive tuberculin skin tests for *M. tuberculosis* in health care workers in Hospital A. This statement is based on certain assumptions: (1) After further evaluation of the problem, the majority of the new infections are all in direct-care employees, specifically the nursing staff. (2) The rate of positive tuberculin skin tests (TST) last year

EXHIBIT 8.1
Population Health and Program Planning Websites

Population Health Websites

www.cdc.gov
http://www.phac-aspc.gc.ca/ph-sp/impact-repercussions/hiatp2.php
www.commissiononhealth.org
www.healthypeople.gov
http://www.gapminder.org/
http://www.inequality.org/
http://www.thelaststraw.ca/
http://www.countyhealthrankings.org/
http://www.nytimes.com/interactive/2011/03/06/weekinreview/20110306-
    happiness.html?ref=weekinreview
www.carecontinuum.org
www.thecommunityguide.org/about/glossary.html
http://www.iom.edu/~/media/Files/Report%20Files/2003/Unequal-Treatment-
    Confronting-Racial-and-Ethnic-Disparities-in-Health-Care/Disparitieshc
    providers8pgFINAL.pdf
http://www.unnaturalcauses.org/

Program Planning Websites

www.cdc.gov
http://wonder.cdc.gov/
http://wonder.cdc.gov/TB.html
http://www.thecommunityguide.org/index.html
http://www.doh.state.fl.us/compass/documents/Healthy%20People%20
    Toolkit.pdf
http://www.cancer.gov/cancertopics/cancerlibrary/theory.pdf
http://www.health.gov/healthypeople/state/toolkit
http://www.healthypeople.gov/2020/implementing/default.aspx
http://www.cdc.gov/healthyplaces/hia.htm
http://www.healthypeople.gov/2010/
http://assessnow.info/
http://www.healthypeople.gov/2010/state/toolkit/default.htm
http://www.cdc.gov/CDCForYou/healthcare_providers.html
http://www.cdc.gov/CDCForYou/researchers.html

---

is known and the number of new positive skin tests is known in the workers
who were not infected last year. For example, if 10 of 1,000 employees tested
positive last year, the prevalence of infection was 1%. A 30% increase this year
would mean that 13 new infections occurred in the 990 employees who did
not test positive last year. (3) Let's also assume that these new positive TSTs
are in employees who were employed at the hospital during the previous year
and had negative TSTs during the screening one year ago. One could suspect,
then, that the employees' risk for exposure to *M. tuberculosis* has increased

Program Development and Evaluation

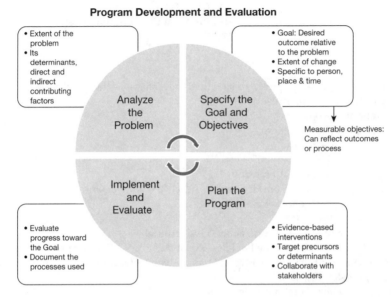

- Extent of the problem
- Its determinants, direct and indirect contributing factors

Analyze the Problem

Specify the Goal and Objectives

- Goal: Desired outcome relative to the problem
- Extent of change
- Specific to person, place & time

Measurable objectives: Can reflect outcomes or process

Implement and Evaluate

Plan the Program

- Evaluate progress toward the Goal
- Document the processes used

- Evidence-based interventions
- Target precursors or determinants
- Collaborate with stakeholders

FIGURE 8.4
Elements of the Program Development and Evaluation Process.
Developed by Deanna E. Grimes DrPH, RN.

and this exposure is more likely to have come from the hospital rather than the community.

Assuming that the analysis of the problem in Figure 8.3 is realistic and based on real information concerning the situation in Hospital A, an APN or anyone responsible for employee health can develop intervention programs to improve infection control practices. Such programs could be to improve the availability, training, and fit of the N95 masks, or to add an isolation room in the Emergency Department. Once again, the CDC Guidelines would help here. The primary question is: How should the APN evaluate whether the interventions were successful? Clearly, the answer is whether the prevalence of new infections in direct-care staff next year, as measured by positive TSTs in staff who were negative this year, has decreased. Ideally, the prevalence rate would be 0% or, at least, less than the previous 1%.

As anyone who has tried to bring about change in any population knows, the ideal does not always occur. What if there is not a decrease in new TB infections, as measured by TST conversions, in direct-care staff in Hospital A after one year of the improved infection control program? Or what if there is some decrease but not as much as expected? First, go back to the analysis of the problem. Is it possible that a major contributing factor was overlooked? For example, has there been such a rapid increase in infections in the community that staff may be exposed outside the hospital? Or is it possible that the number of patients admitted to the hospital with non-symptomatic active TB disease that is undiagnosed has increased substantially? Have any other contributing factors been overlooked when planning the intervention?

Second, was the goal realistic? What is the average prevalence rate for new infections in other direct-care hospital staff working in the same region as Hospital A, in the state, and in the nation? Maybe the small decrease in new infections in Hospital A is comparable to the situation in other hospitals and that the original goal exceeded the standard at the time.

Third, were all of the infection control plans implemented as designed? For example, were new N95 masks ordered and made available on all patient care units in a timely manner? Were all staff fitted appropriately for the masks and trained to use them? Are staff members using the masks as they were trained to do? Was the isolation room in the Emergency Department available for use in a timely manner? Are patients with respiratory symptoms being triaged to the isolation area as soon as they arrive at the emergency area?

There are additional general factors, sometimes called intervening variables, to consider when desired outcomes in a population are not achieved within the desired timeframe. Has something in the population changed, increasing their risk or making them more vulnerable? Have they aged or has their health status declined? For example, one might investigate whether the job of the direct-care staff has changed such that their potential exposure to *M. tuberculosis* has increased.

Also look at the environment for possible change that has increased the risk to staff. Has the ratio of patients to staff increased so much as to preclude staff using adequate infection control practices? Is it possible that patients, who have been inadequately treated for active tuberculosis disease and now have multidrug resistant tuberculosis (MDRTB), are being admitted to the hospital? Another possibility to consider is whether patients are sicker at admission because of changes in their insurance coverage, and, therefore, are expelling more bacteria in mucous droplets when they cough.

The new information learned from the evaluation can then influence further analysis of the problem and further planning, as depicted in Figure 8.4. The process of improving the health of populations is not unlike that of improving the health of an individual patient. The process begins with an understanding of basic social, behavioral, biologic, and physical environmental concepts influencing individuals and populations. One then proceeds to assess and diagnose health problems in both individuals and populations. Part of the diagnosis is to quantify a problem by comparing the characteristics of the problem with a standard. The next step is to analyze the problem by applying scientific evidence and direct observation of the conditions surrounding the problem in order to highlight the factors contributing to the problem. This step provides direction for the intervention to prevent progression of the problem. One then determines the outcome that is desired with respect to the problem and plans interventions to achieve that goal. If the goal is not reached, the problem is further assessed and analyzed and the planning circuit continued. If the goal is achieved, the individual patient or the population experiences a higher level of health.

REFERENCES

American Association of Colleges of Nursing. (2006). *The essentials of doctoral education for Advanced Practice Nursing.* Retrieved from www.aacn. nche.edu

Centers for Disease Control and Prevention. (2005). National Center for HIV, STD, and TB Prevention. Guidelines for preventing the transmission of Mycobacterium tuberculosis in health-care settings 2005. *Morbidity and Mortality Weekly Report, 54*(RR17), 1–144.

Glouberman, S., & Miller, J. (2003). Evolution of the determinants of health, health policy, and health information systems in Canada. *American Journal of Public Health, 93*, 388–392.

Turnock, B. J. (2009). *Public health: What it is and how it works* (4th ed.). Sudbury, MA: Jones and Bartlett Publishers.

U.S. Department of Health and Human Services. (2001). *Healthy people 2010: Understanding and improving health.* Retrieved from http://www.healthypeople. gov/Document/tableofcontents.htm#under

U.S. Department of Health and Human Services. (2002). *Healthy People 2010* (2nd ed.). Washington, DC: U.S. Government Printing Office.

U.S. Department of Health and Human Services. (2009). *Healthy people 2020.* Retrieved from http://www.healthypeople.gov/2020/about/DOHAbout.aspx

U.S. Department of Health and Human Services. (ND). *Healthy people 2010: A systematic approach.* Retrieved from http://www.healthypeople.gov/2010/Document/html/uih/uih_2.htm#deter

NINE

Evaluating Health Care Teams

Joanne V. Hickey

*"None of us is as smart as all of us.... We all know that cooperation
and collaboration grow more important every day. A shrinking world in
which technological and political complexity increase at an accelerated
rate offers fewer and fewer arenas in which individual action suffices."*

Warren Bennis, 1996

INTRODUCTION

The current literature overwhelmingly exalts the value of teams—in particular, interdisciplinary health care teams—as the primary way to achieve better
patient outcomes. As one delves into the literature to find and examine the
supporting evidence for such a claim, the results are surprising. What one
finds are mostly descriptions, observations, case studies, and expert opinion
reports, but few well-designed investigations of health care teams. The work
of teams is complex, and the magnitude of complexity increases with greater
numbers of team members, the focus of the work, and contextual environmental factors. Teams are dynamic with complex internal and external interactions.
Internal interactions are within the team and include member-to-member and
member-to-team interactions. External sources include interactions with the
patent/family, other teams, the organization, elements of the organization,
oversight committees, and the overall health care delivery system.

Teams are ever changing as they undergo multiple transitions in their
work and goals responding to the needs of patients, organizations, and the
health care system. A onetime snapshot of a team does little to capture the
immense complexity and dynamics of the team, which suggests the need to
study teams over time, thus creating multiple snapshots. In addition, current

research methodologies are generally ineffective at enlightening investigators about the complex interactive processes and outcomes of teams. Most studies provide insight about a few variables of interest by reporting relationships among selected variables, but do not address causality. The state of the science on health care teams is "messy," although it provides some direction for evaluation of teams.

The purpose of this chapter is to provide the reader with background information about health care teams, including the theoretical/conceptual basis, types, development, functions, and outcomes of teams as well as core competencies for interprofessions collaborative practice. This information serves as a basis for better understanding teams and as possible foci for evaluation. It also provides a framework for evaluating teams.

WHAT IS A TEAM AND TEAMWORK?

Both teams and teamwork have many definitions. Lorimer and Manion (1996) define a team as "a small number of consistent people committed to a relevant shared purpose, with common performance goals, complementary and overlapping skills, and a common approach to their work." According to Xyrichis and Ream (2008), teamwork is "a dynamic process involving two or more healthcare professionals with complementary backgrounds and skills, sharing common health goals and exercising concerted physical and mental effort in assessing, planning, or evaluating patient care." Teamwork occurs by using a number of strategies such as interdependent collaboration, open communications, shared decision making, and generated value-added patient, organizational, and staff outcomes (Xyrichis & Ream, 2008).

Teams can be further classified as *conventional teams*, which is defined as those teams whose members interact through traditional meetings and consultation. The electronic era has fostered the development of *electronic teams* whose members interact through new communications processes augmented by electronic technology such as the Internet. Web-based tools using multifunctional software application enable teamwork to occur at anytime and anywhere (Heintz & Origgi, 2005; Wiecha & Pollard, 2004).

TYPES OF TEAMS

In health care, the teams of greatest interest are the teams classified as multidisciplinary, interdisciplinary, interprofessional, and transdisciplinary. Table 9.1 includes terms used in describing teams. Choi and Pak (2006) addressed the development and clarity of terminology in a comprehensive review of terminology and suggested that these terms reflect a continuum. Although there continues to be some confusion about the definitions of terms, the following definitions are provided as a basis for discussion.

TABLE 9.1

Definitions Related to Health Care Teams

Term	Definition
Collaboration	Cooperatively working together, sharing responsibility for solving problems and making decisions to formulate and carry out plans for patient care (Baggs & Schmitt, 1988, p. 145; Baggs et al., 1999). A complex process through which relationships are developed among health care professionals so that they effectively interact and work together for the mutual goal of safe and quality patient care (Freshman, Rubino, & Chassiakos, 2010, p. 110).
Interdisciplinary collaboration	Interdisciplinary collaboration is an interpersonal process that facilitates the achievement of goals that cannot be reached when individual professionals act individually.
Leadership	The ability to coordinate the activities of team members and teams by managing the resources available to team members and facilitating team performance by communicating plans, providing information about team performance through debriefs, and providing support to team members when needed (TeamSTEPPS Instructor Guide Glossary, 2011).
Team effectiveness	The degree to which team goals and objectives are successfully met.
Team mental models	The shared and organized understanding and mental representation of knowledge or beliefs relevant to key elements of the team's task environment (Klimoski & Mohammed, 1994).
Team processes	Interdependent acts of members that convert inputs into outputs through cognitive, verbal, and behavioral activities directed toward organizing task work to achieve collective goals. Task work involves what the team is doing, and reflects skill and member competence. By contrast, teamwork describes how they do it, and relies on higher-level behaviors such as the ability to direct, align, communicate, negotiate, and monitor task work (Marks et al., 2001).
Value	Value has different meanings in different contexts. Value in health care is expressed as the physical health and sense of well-being achieved related to the cost (IOM Roundtable on Evidence-Based Medicine, 2008).

Multidisciplinary refers to a team where members of different disciplines assess or treat patients independently and then share the information with each other (Sorrells-Jones, 1997). Members of different disciplines contribute to the care of a patient, but do so independently and without knowledge of the overall specific goals or what other team members are doing. Although written documentation of care is available from each provider, it is a "silo" approach to care, with each provider "doing her or his own thing." Coordination, continuity of care, and a comprehensive approach to the achievement of common goals are lacking.

Interdisciplinary describes a deeper level of collaboration in which processes such as development of a plan of care or evaluation occur jointly, with professionals of different disciplines pooling their knowledge in an independent way (Sorrells-Jones, 1997). When the term interdisciplinary is attached to the term practice, then *interdisciplinary practice* refers to people with distinct disciplinary education and training working together for a common purpose through different but complementary contributions to patient-focused care (Leathard, 1994). In current practice, an interdisciplinary model of practice and care is considered best practice. The model is used across the continuum of care including intensive care units, long-term care facilities, geriatric acute and chronic care units, transitional care units, and community-based clinics. Although based on an interdisciplinary model, the interpretation and implementation of the model has great variability across settings and facilities.

Transdisciplinary is a specific form of interdisciplinarity in which boundaries between and beyond disciplines are transcended and knowledge and perspectives from different scientific disciplines as well as non-scientific sources are integrated (Vrije University Amsterdam, 2005). Transdisciplinary is the newest term in the disciplinarity nomenclature and is undergoing the process of consensus building around a definition. The prefix "trans" means to go across something. By going across, beyond, and over disciplinary boundaries, a process emerges to assemble the disciplines in new ways and to recombine disciplinary knowledge and information for the creating of new knowledge (Choi & Pak, 2006). There is great interest concerning transdisciplinary teams because of the complexity of current problems and the belief that only transdisciplinary thinking and problem solving can adequately address these challenges. It is transdisciplinary teams of molecular scientists, biological engineers, geneticists, ethicists, and others that are needed to solve such complex questions related to stem cell and personal health issues (Massachusetts Institute of Technology, 2011).

Interprofessional describes the interactions among individual professionals who may represent a particular discipline or branch of knowledge, but who additionally bring their unique educational background, experiences, values, roles, and identities to the process of working across health care professions to cooperate, collaborate, communicate, and integrate care in teams to ensure that care is continuous and reliable. Each professional may possess some shared or overlapping knowledge, skills, abilities, competencies, and roles with other professionals with whom he or she collaborates (Ash & Miller, 2010; Institute of Medicine [IOM], 2003). Some argue that interprofessional is a subset of intradisciplinary, while others say it is limited only to the work of members of a discipline, which is described as a profession. The limitation excludes anyone who is not classified as a "professional" and thus excludes potential providers of information and knowledge to the work at hand including the patient and family, and it is counterintuitive to patient-centered care.

In contemporary practice the pursuit of multiple disciplinarity and teamwork is important for several reasons including the following (Choi & Pak, 2006):

- To resolve real-world problems
- To resolve complex problems
- To provide different perspectives about a problem
- To create a comprehensive prospective theory-based hypothesis for research
- To develop consensus around clinical definitions and guidelines for complex diseases and conditions
- To provide comprehensive services such as health care and health education

CORE COMPETENCIES FOR INTERPROFESSIONAL COLLABORATIVE PRACTICE

The Core Competencies for Interprofessional Collaborative Practice is the work of the Interprofessional Education Collaborative (IPEC, 2011), which represents six national professional education associations (nursing, osteopathic medicine, pharmacy, dentistry, medicine, and public health). The report provides key definitions and principles that guided the identification of core interprofessional competencies and eight reasons why it is important to agree on a core set of competencies across the professions. The interprofessional collaborative practice competency domains include the following:

Competency Domain 1: Values/Ethics for Interprofessional Practice
Competency Domain 2: Roles and Responsibilities
Competency Domain 3: Interprofessional Communication
Competency Domain 4: Teams and Teamwork

Table 9.2 includes a general competency statement for each domain followed by the specific competencies (IPEC, 2011, pp. 16–25). These domains and competencies are useful for the APN to consider in evaluating team functionality and team performance.

TABLE 9.2

Interprofessional Collaborative Practice Competency Domain, Competency Statements, and Specific Competencies for Each Domain

---

Competency Domain 1: Values/Ethics for Interprofessional Practice

General Competency Statement-VE. Work with individuals of other professions to maintain a climate of mutual respect and shared values.

Specific Values/Ethics Competencies:

VE1. Place the interests of patients and populations at the center of interprofessional health care delivery.

VE2. Respect the dignity and privacy of patients while maintaining confidentiality in the delivery of team-based care.

VE3. Embrace the cultural diversity and individual differences that characterize patients, populations, and the health care team.

VE4. Respect the unique cultures, values, roles/responsibilities, and expertise of other health professions.

VE5. Work in cooperation with those who receive care, those who provide care, and others who contribute to or support the delivery of prevention and health services.

VE6. Develop a trusting relationship with patients, families, and other team members (CIHC, 2010).

VE7. Demonstrate high standards of ethical conduct and quality of care in one's contributions to team-based care.

VE8. Manage ethical dilemmas specific to interprofessional patient/population centered care situations.

VE9. Act with honesty and integrity in relationships with patients, families, and other team members.

VE10. Maintain competence in one's own profession appropriate to scope of practice.

Competency Domain 2: Roles and Responsibilities

General Competency Statement-RR. Use the knowledge of one's own role and those of other professions to appropriately assess and address the healthcare needs of the patients and populations served.

Specific Roles/Responsibilities Competencies:

RR1. Communicate one's roles and responsibilities clearly to patients, families, and other professionals.

RR2. Recognize one's limitations in skills, knowledge, and abilities.

RR3. Engage diverse healthcare professionals who complement one's own professional expertise, as well as associated resources, to develop strategies to meet specific patient care needs.

RR4. Explain the roles and responsibilities of other care providers and how the team works together to provide care.

(continued)

TABLE 9.2 (*continued*)

RR5. Use the full scope of knowledge, skills, and abilities of available health professionals and healthcare workers to provide care that is safe, timely, efficient, effective, and equitable.

RR6. Communicate with team members to clarify each member's responsibility in executing components of a treatment plan or public health intervention.

RR7. Forge interdependent relationships with other professions to improve care and advance learning.

RR8. Engage in continuous professional and interprofessional development to enhance team performance.

RR9. Use unique and complementary abilities of all members of the team to optimize patient care.

Competency Domain 3: Interprofessional Communication

General Competency Statement-CC. Communicate with patients, families, communities, and other health professionals in a responsive and responsible manner that supports a team approach to the maintenance of health and the treatment of disease.

Specific Interprofessional Communication Competencies:

CC1. Choose effective communication tools and techniques, including information systems and communication technologies, to facilitate discussions and interactions that enhance team function.

CC2. Organize and communicate information with patients, families, and healthcare team members in a form that is understandable, avoiding discipline-specific terminology when possible.

CC3. Express one's knowledge and opinions to team members involved in patient care with confidence, clarity, and respect, working to ensure common understanding of information and treatment and care decisions.

CC4. Listen actively, and encourage ideas and opinions of other team members.

CC5. Give timely, sensitive, instructive feedback to others about their performance on the team, responding respectfully as a team member to feedback from others.

CC6. Use respectful language appropriate for a given difficult situation, crucial conversation, or interprofessional conflict.

CC7. Recognize how one's own uniqueness, including experience level, expertise, culture, power, and hierarchy within the healthcare team, contributes to effective communication, conflict resolution, and positive interprofessional working relationships (University of Toronto, 2008).

CC8. Communicate consistently the importance of teamwork in patient-centered and community-focused care.

(*continued*)

TABLE 9.2

Interprofessional Collaborative Practice Competency Domain, Competency Statements, and Specific Competencies for Each Domain (*continued*)

Competency Domain 4: Teams and Teamwork

General Competency Statement-TT. Apply relationship-building values and the principles of team dynamics to perform effectively in different team roles to plan and deliver patient-Zpopulation-centered care that is safe, timely, efficient, effective, and equitable.

Specific Team and Teamwork Competencies:

TT1. Describe the process of team development and the roles and practices of effective teams.

TT2. Develop consensus on the ethical principles to guide all aspects of patient care and team work.

TT3. Engage other health professionals—appropriate to the specific care situation—in shared patient-centered problem-solving.

TT4. Integrate the knowledge and experience of other professions—appropriate to the specific care situation—to inform care decisions, while respecting patient and community values and priorities/ preferences for care.

TT5. Apply leadership practices that support collaborative practice and team effectiveness.

TT6. Engage self and others to constructively manage disagreements about values, roles, goals, and actions that arise among healthcare professionals and with patients and families.

TT7. Share accountability with other professions, patients, and communities for outcomes relevant to prevention and health care.

TT8. Reflect on individual and team performance for individual, as well as team, performance improvement.

TT9. Use process improvement strategies to increase the effectiveness of interprofessional teamwork and team-based care.

TT10. Use available evidence to inform effective teamwork and team-based practices.

TT11. Perform effectively on teams and in different team roles in a variety of settings.

DEVELOPMENT OF TEAMS

Team development is usually regarded as an informal process by which group members attempt to create effective social structures and work processes on their own (Kozlowski & Ilgen, 2006). A number of team developmental process models are available, but perhaps the most commonly cited model is that of Tuckman (1965). The model initially included the four stages of forming, storming, norming, and performing; a fifth stage, adjourning, was later added (Tuckman & Jensen, 1977). These are the stages that small groups are likely to go through as they come together and begin to function (Smith, 2005). The *forming stage* is described as a time of orientation through testing. The testing helps to identify boundaries of both interpersonal and task behaviors. Interpersonal work is around the establishment of dependency relationships with leaders, other group members, or pre-existing standards. In the *storming stage* there is conflict and polarization around interpersonal issues with concomitant emotional response around tasks. These behaviors serve as resistance to group influence and task requirements. In the *norming stage* resistance is overcome because of the development of in-group feeling and cohesiveness, evolution of new standards, and adoption of new roles. Personal opinions are expressed. The *performing stage* is characterized by effective interpersonal structures to accomplish the work, roles become flexible and functional, and group energy is channeled into getting the work done. Structural issues have been resolved and an effective structure supports group work. Finally, in the *adjourning stage* the focus is on dissolution or termination of roles, the completion of tasks, and reduction of dependency. Particularly if unplanned, the process of adjourning can be stressful with a component of mourning related to individual losses.

The following factors facilitate teams to progress through the stages of team development as a high performance team (Ash & Miller, 2010):

- Shared purpose, goals, and commitment of team members
- Mutual trust among team members
- Recognition and value of the unique role or skills which each member brings
- High performance in level of skills, ability, and practice
- Clear understanding of roles and the responsibility and accountability of each team member to meet the goals
- A work culture and environment that supports team and collaborative processes
- Collective cognitive responsibility and shared decision making

The Tuckman (1965) model of the development sequence of small groups is a linear model that has stood the test of time although some have challenged the linearity in favor of models that reflect the fluctuations of groups. There does appear to be general support that small groups tend to follow a fairly predictable developmental path (Smith, 2011). From the perspective of evaluation, the Tuckman model can provide insight into group process and achievement of outcomes. The developmental stage of the group is one variable in understanding and evaluating groups.

THEORETICAL PERSPECTIVE OF TEAMS

Most of the literature on teams is opinion/expert commentary, descriptive, and case studies. The literature about teams in general and health teams specifically is voluminous. Teams can be viewed from multiple perspectives. Since the 1950s, the social, organizational, and business/management sciences have investigated teams from a variety of discipline specific perspectives resulting in an overwhelming number of theoretical frameworks to view teams. A number of theories have been developed with a focus on teams including how teams are organized, how they work, and how they achieve outcomes. One can evaluate teams based on group dynamics, effectiveness, efficiency, interpersonal communications, satisfaction, and outcomes. A brief discussion of the theoretical basis of teams is useful to better understand the multiple lenses that can be used to examine and evaluate teams.

Team behavior through the conceptualization of group processes was strongly influenced by sociological studies of hierarchical differentiation (Ingersoll & Schmitt, 2004). The primary focus of research was on the group's social structure and its influence on team communications and problem solving (Feiger & Schmitt, 1979). Another example of a sociological view is the theory of Groupthink (Janis, 1982), defined as a condition in which highly cohesive groups in "hot" decision situations display excessive levels of concurrence seeking that suppresses critical inquiry and result in faulty decision making. Farrell, Heineman, and Schmitt (1986), Farrell, Heinemann, and Schmitt (1988), and Farrell, Schmitt, and Heinemann (1988, 2001) proposed guidelines to counteract poor team decision making processes with the following: (1) emphasize open, honest, and direct communications; (2) facilitate team development through orientation of new team members and team retreats; (3) focus on the team's mission statement, goals, policies, and procedures; (4) acknowledge effective individual and team work; and (5) identify team processes that lead to poor decision making with a focus on finding more effective decision making processes (Ingersoll & Schmitt, 2004).

The organizational literature has focused on theories such as high-reliability organizations (HRO), organizational structure, team performance, and learning organizations. Team structure is the fundamental characteristic of teams, and structure includes size, membership, leadership, identification, and distribution. Weick and Roberts (1993) examined HROs that espoused to be nearly error free operations. They found that these organizations integrate highly developed mental models and processes that all members follow, which are a reflection of overlapping knowledge and performance standards. Another example of organizational theory is that of learning organizations. Senge (1990), in addressing systems thinking, notes that team learning is vital because teams, not individuals, are the fundamental learning unit in modern organizations. Unless a team can learn, the organization cannot learn. Excellence in any organization is not a specific arrival destination; rather, great organizations are always in a state of learning to become better or worse by expanding their capacity to create their futures.

Microsystem theory and macrosystem theory are other paths of organizational investigation. A microsystem refers to the next coherent organizational level above individuals, typically a small team of people working together as one unit to get jobs done (Nelson, Batalden, & Godfrey, 2007, pp. 206–209). In aviation, the microsystem is the flight crew and air traffic controllers. In health care, it is the health care team. Microsystem theory focuses on the front-line component of service delivery. Nelson et al. (2002) used a qualitative methodology to investigate high performance clinical microsystems. The researchers identified characteristics across sites that led to excellent systemic outcomes. These characteristics include: leadership and the culture of the microsystems; macro-organizational support of the microsystem; a focus on patients and staff; interdependence of care teams; easy access to information and information technology; a focus on process improvement; and high level performance patterns (Nelson et al., 2002).

As described in Chapter 1, a macrosystem refers to the overarching structure above the microsystem such as the organization or the system. A macrosystem includes the policies, procedures, culture, and leadership that oversee the microsystems. Interactions between the microsystem and macrosystem affect performance and outcomes at both levels.

The literature on health care teams reflects a mounting body of knowledge that supports superior outcomes from health care teams as compared to an individual practitioner. The limited integrative reviews that have been published provide insight into the development of knowledge about health care teams. Halstead (1976) reviewed ten studies that emphasized chronic illness and rehabilitation. He categorized the literature into the three areas of opinion articles, description of programs, and investigations of the effectiveness of team care. Most of the publications fell into the first two categories and described patient functional outcomes. They did not say if the teams were effective. A second review examined the research on effectiveness of interdisciplinary team (Schmitt 2001; Schmitt, Farrell, & Heinemann, 1988) and generally concluded that teams improve functional outcomes although there were also mixed findings. The studies reviewed did not examine greater use of resources, cost variables, or multidimensional factors of team relationships and their impact on care.

Schofield and Amodeo (1999) reviewed the education, psychology, sociology, and medical databases to identify reports on interdisciplinary teams. Of the 138 articles reviewed, 55 were descriptive addressing some component of interdisciplinary teams; team processes or the influence of data on process or outcomes were not examined. Another 51 articles described interdisciplinary team processes, but did not provide supporting data. Although research based, another 21 articles examined a variety of variables and their effect on the team. Finally, another group of 11 articles were described as outcome based because research methods were used to assess the impact of an interdisciplinary team on selected outcomes other than team functioning. In summarizing the literature, Schofield and Amodeo (1999) noted the following: 1) although the literature endorses the team model and assumes the value of interdisciplinary teams, there is little evidence to evaluate team effectiveness or impact; and 2) the absence of well-conceived conceptual models of interdisciplinary teamwork or models to assess components of the interdisciplinary process makes it difficult to drawn any reliable conclusions.

A Cochrane systematic review addressed interprofessional collaboration practice and health outcomes. The review suggests that practice-based interprofessional collaboration can improve health care processes and outcomes, but because of the limitations of the literature (e.g., small number of studies, sample sizes, problems with conceptualization and measurement of collaboration, and heterogeneity of interventions and settings), it was not possible to draw generalizable conclusions about the key elements of interprofessional collaboration and its effectiveness (Zwarenstein, Goldman, & Reeves, 2009). More studies and methodological rigor were recommended to better understand interprofessional collaboration.

The need for greater interprofessional collaboration has been emphasized since the 1970s (IOM, 2010). A growing body of research has begun to highlight the potential for collaboration among teams composed of diverse individuals to generate successful solutions in complex, knowledge-driven problems (Paulus & Nijstad, 2003; Posano & Verganti, 2008; Singh & Fleming, 2010; Wuchty, Jones, & Uzzi, 2007). Researchers have also emphasized the importance of building interprofessional teams and establishing collaborative cultures to identify and sustain continuous improvement of the quality of care (Kim, Barnato, Angus, Fleisher, & Kahn 2010; Knaus, 1986; Pronovost et al., 2008). Interest in collaboration as a concept integral to interdisciplinary practice was explored. Ingersoll and Schmitt (2004) noted that this basic shift in conceptualization is important because it highlights the concept of collaboration in the delivery of care among diverse health professions.

Beginning in the late 1980s, Baggs and Schmitt (1988) investigated collaboration and interdisciplinary teams within health care organizations. *Collaboration* was defined as "cooperatively working together, sharing responsibility for solving problems and making decisions to formulate and carry out plans for patient care" (Baggs & Schmitt, 1988, p. 145). An aim of collaboration is to coordinate care and improve patient outcomes. Baggs and Schmitt (1997) focused much of their early work on physician-nurse collaboration in critical care settings. Concurrently, Knaus, Draper, Wagner, and Zimmerman (1986) developed the Acute Physiology and Chronic Health Evaluation (APACHE) score to predict mortality in intensive care unit (ICU) patients. They also observed that high levels of interdisciplinary practice and coordination contributed to better patient outcomes.

Using a nurse-physician questionnaire to evaluate perceptions of the multiple dimensions of the processes of care in ICUs, Shortell et al. (1992, 1994) noted that communication, leadership, coordination, and conflict management were related to better technical care, meeting of family needs, and decreased length of stay. Twenty-five ICUs were investigated in a national study conducted by Mitchell, Shannon, Cain, and Hegyvary (1996). Flow of information characteristic of interdisciplinary collaboration was associated with better staff perceptions of unit conflict management, collaboration, staff quality, and quality of care, but it was not associated with better clinical outcomes. Other evidence of the benefits of teamwork has emerged and includes increased learning and development of people and organizations, better utilization of resources and planning, minimization of unnecessary costs, improved job performance work quality, increased discussion among participants, networking, professional development, and positive effect on career (Choi & Pak, 2006).

Andretta (2010) conducted an observational study of teams using qualitative methods of observation and categorization to inform a model of team development strategies. The results suggested that health care teams may be more complicated than non-health care teams. Team models with associated competencies identified from other professions may not transfer completely to health care. Further, a single model to inform best practices for health care team development may not adequately address the specific performance challenges of each team type found in health care, thus requiring a variety of different strategies to optimize team performance.

Many other studies have examined interdisciplinary teams and collaboration in relationship to patient outcomes in a variety of settings such as nursing homes, long-term care facilities, acute/critical care units, rehabilitation, and primary care, as well as with specific populations such as geriatrics, the chronically ill, and others (Boaro, Fancott, Baker, Velji, & Andreoli, 2010; Boult et al., 2009; Famadas et al., 2008; Korner, 2010; Meier & Beresford, 2010; Neumann et al., 2010; Pezzin et al., 2011; Pyne et al., 2011; Reader, Fin, Mearns, & Cuthbertson, 2009; Rocco, Scher, Basberg, Yalamanchi, & Baker-Genaw, 2011). What is clear is that little is known empirically about interdisciplinary teams and collaboration including team effectiveness and impact on health care delivery. Health care teams are complex dynamic entities working in complex dynamic environments. Marks, Mathieu, and Zaccaro (2001) noted that the framework of team processes and outcomes are multidimensional, and team behavior is constantly changing. The changing nature of a team and team member behavior is tempered by the developmental level of the team and the work of the team that transitions between existing goals and new goals including evolving processes. As previously noted, a single snapshot of a team provides little information in understanding how teams work in the achievement of outcomes. Therefore, new models to investigate teams are needed if theoretical frameworks based on evidence are to be useful in health care delivery.

Nurse researchers have tried to untangle the role and contributions of the nurse in teams and have found it to be methodologically challenging.

The Magnet® Recognition Program, administered by the American Nurses Credentialing Center, is a credential for nursing excellence awarded to health care facilities and is based on extensive self-review that demonstrates achievement of established criteria of nursing excellence that achieves outstanding patient outcomes. A health care organization that chooses to seek this credential begins the magnet journey to create a sustainable culture and work environment that supports excellence in professional nursing practice. The initial qualitative research that was foundational to creating the Magnet Program was conducted by McClure, Poulin, Sovie, and Wandelt (1983). Participant hospitals were nominated as places that were able to attract and retain professional nurses. The study included 41 hospitals representative of the all regions of the country. Among the characteristics identified as essential in these facilities was good interdisciplinary relationships, defined as interdisciplinary effort and shared decision making, along with a sense of mutual respect exhibited among all disciplines. Among the 14 forces of magnetism outlined in the current Magnet model, interdisciplinary relationships continues to be a force within the category of exemplary professional practice.

Using a structure-process-outcome framework to examine research supporting interdisciplinary relationships, Reid-Ponte, Creta, and Joy (2011) suggest that there is limited research evidence supporting the premise that effectively led, collaborative, interdisciplinary care teams improve patient care processes and outcomes (Boyle & Kochinda, 2004; Cowan et al., 2006; DeChairo-Marino, Jordon-Marsh, Traiger, & Saulo, 2001; Grumbach & Bodenheimer, 2004; Horbar, Plsek, Leahy, & Ford, 2004; Houldin, Naylor, & Haller, 2004). They go on to say that practice environment research supports the idea that the more mutually collaborative and respectful a team is perceived, the higher the quality of care they perceive is delivered (Aiken, Clarke, Cheung, Sloane, & Silber 2004; Aiken, Clarke, & Sloane, 2002; Friese, Lake, Aiken, Silver, & Sochalski, 2008).

Lemieux-Charles and McGuire (2006) reviewed health care team effectiveness literature from 1985 to 2004 and distinguish among intervention studies that compare team with usual (nonteam) care, intervention studies that examine the impact of team redesign on team effectiveness, and field studies that explore relationships amongteam context, structure, processes, and outcomes. Using an Integrated Team Effectiveness Model (ITEM) to summarize research findings and to identify gaps in the literature, their analysis suggested that the type and diversity of clinical expertise involved in team decision making largely accounts for improvements in patient care and organizational effectiveness. Collaboration, conflict resolution, participation, and cohesion are most likely to influence staff satisfaction and perceived team effectiveness. The studies examined here underscore the importance of considering the contexts in which teams are embedded.

These examples offer a glimpse of some theoretical frameworks from disciplines both outside and inside of health care to provide a foundation for viewing health care teams, as well as insight into the investigational paths pursued. Research is slowly evolving regarding teams and interdisciplinary practice teams and how they affect patient outcomes. Table 9.3 provides a list of variables related to health care teams that have been investigated. These variable have been extracted from studies cited in the chapter and personal experience, and have been organized into arbitrary categories as a way to organize them. Each category is mutually exclusive from the other categories, although variables from a number of categories may be examined during a particular evaluation. From a cursory review of the list, it is clear that there are multiple perspectives that can be used to examine and evaluate teams.

TABLE 9.3
Perspectives for Evaluating Health Care Team

Group Process Perspective
- Interactions of team members
- Accomplishment of tasks
- Engagement in team activities
- Engagement in team development activities
- Decision-making processes (e.g., shared, hierarchal)
- Competition between and among members
- Team norms

Communications Perspective
- Open, honest, and direct communications
- Constructive feedback
- Effective conflict resolution

Cohesiveness Perspective
- Commitment to mutual purpose
- Understanding and commitment to team mission, goals, policies, and procedures
- Orientation of new members
- Supporting of team members
- Shared team mental model

High Performance Perspective
- Shared vision
- Clear responsibilities
- Mutual respect
- Trust
- Cohesiveness
- Expectation of accountability of all members for outcomes
- Appreciation of expertise and contribution of each discipline
- Collaboration
- Interdisciplinary working together
- Individual and team effectiveness
- Shared decision making
- Team members supportive of team decisions and each other
- Use common mental models
- Coordination of care

Structural Perspective
- Vertical versus horizontal
- Shared versus hierarchal authority
- Hierarchal leadership
- Make-up of the team (e.g., disciplines represented) and how this contributes to outcomes

(continued)

TABLE 9.3
Perspectives for Evaluating Health Care Team (*continued*)

Leadership Perspective

- Hierarchal versus shared leadership
- Interchange of leadership and followership
- Person with the most knowledge for particular project leads
- Leadership development opportunities available to all members
- Organizational support for team

Individual Team Member Perspective

- Values
- Attitudes
- Autonomy
- Motivation
- Personal and professional development
- Confidence building
- Self monitoring
- Emotional intelligence

Team Development Perspective

- Crew resource management
- Culture of learning
- Individual and group competency

Satisfaction Perspective

- Patient/family satisfaction with team
- Individual team members satisfied with team
- Others external to the team such as employer, administrator, or funder

Patient Outcome Perspective

- Length of stay
- Mortality
- Morbidity/complications
- Functionality (e.g., social, intellectual, activities of daily living [ADLs], instrumental ADLs)
- Cost of care
- Service utilization

Safety and Quality Perspective

- Culture of blame versus quality improvement
- Root cause analysis

BARRIERS TO TEAMS

In the health care arena, there are many barriers to establishing and maintaining high performance teams. Some barriers cut across all practice areas while others are specific to particular areas of practice and environments. Barriers to interprofessional collaboration include the following (Ash & Miller, 2010):

- Gender, power, socialization, education, status, and cultural differences between professions
- Reimbursement systems and structures that do not reward interprofessional collaboration
- Lack of clarify and understanding about the scope of practice and contributions of each profession to patient care
- Turf protection that is both intradisciplinary and interdisciplinary

■ Local customs and cultures
■ Technical and team competency

Durbin (2006) notes that local customs may be the most difficult barrier to overcome. In addition, resistance comes from many sources such as hospital administration (concern about added cost), unit administrator (change in authority and control), bedside staff (must learn new ways of interacting with a team), and private physicians (altered authority gradient for patient management and decisions). Both technical competency and team competency are necessary to achieve high performance in interdisciplinary teams. Technical competency is based on professional training, education, and experience as well as licensure and certification. Team competency is based on education and the knowledge, skills, and attitude about interdisciplinary work. In addition, competency may be defined differently in each discipline.

FAILURE OF TEAMS

Health care teams are often viewed through the lens of quality and safety. Understanding why and how teams fail is critical to understanding corrective interventions to support high performance teams. Sassou and Reason (1999) reviewed adverse events in the nuclear, aviation, and shipping industries and found the most common cause of error was failure to communicate. The root causes of failure to communicate were authority gradient, excessive professional courtesy, over-trusting, projected confidence, inadequate resources, and poor task management, all of which resulted in a lack of ability to detect both individual and group error. Also noted was that there is a limit to how far any individual can be "perfected" and made "error-proof," and that a much higher limit of quality and safety can be achieved by using a team that spots for each other and works together. Strategies to keep teams and organizations functioning within industry-accepted safety standards have been developed and include crew resource management (CRM), also known as team cooperation training. CRM is used extensively by the military and aviation industry and encompasses a wide range of techniques to enhance communications, situational awareness, problem solving, decision making, teamwork, and making optimal use of all available resources (e.g., equipment, procedures, people) to promote and enhance efficiency of flight operations (TeamSTEPPS, 2011).

INSTRUMENTS

Instruments have been developed to assess teams from a variety of perspectives. In conducting an evaluation of a team, there are some validated instruments that can be used to collect data about variables of interest. The instruments are designed to measure a few domains of interest although no one instrument will meet the needs of all users. On the other hand, in searching for a validated instrument, the evaluator may not find any instrument that is appropriate for the purpose and focus of the evaluation. Examples of available instruments are described in this section to acquaint the reader with a few existing instruments and what they were designed to measure. All of the instruments mentioned have alleged high reliability and validity.

The Collaboration Assessment Tool (Baggs, Ryan, Phelps, Richeson, & Johnson, 1992; Baggs et al., 1997) was developed to measure nurse-physician collaboration in making specific decisions about patient care, as well as provider satisfaction with the decision-making process and the decisions make. The questionnaire was designed to be administered to providers as they deliver care. Another instrument called the Index of Interdisciplinary Collaboration (IIC; Bronstein, 2002) was designed to measure the extent of collaboration between social workers and other professionals from a social work perspective. The IIC can be used to assess these professional interactions with the goal of improved services to clients.

The Department of Veterans Affairs wanted to improve communications within the health care environment and developed the Medical Team Training (MTT) questionnaire to assess organizational culture, communication, teamwork, and awareness of human factors engineering principles. In piloting the instrument to an interdisciplinary group of 384 surgical staff members in six facilities, they found that the MTT was helpful in identifying discrepancies in communication patterns in which surgeons perceived a stronger organizational culture of safety, better communications, and better teamwork than either nurses or anesthesiologists did (Mills, Neily, & Dunn, 2008).

The Healthcare Team Vitality Instrument (HTVI) was developed to assess health care team functioning as it relates to nurses and other licensed and unlicensed personnel working as part of the health care team in inpatient hospital units. The reasons for developing this instrument were twofold: 1) to provide an instrument that assesses the characteristics of registered nurses or perceptions about the characteristics of the organization in which they work in combination with interdisciplinary team function and collaboration; and 2) to provide a short, user-friendly instrument that could be helpful to monitor the impact of changes designed to improve work environments (Upenieks, Lee, Flanagan, & Doebbeling, 2009).

The Mayo High Performance Teamwork Scale (Malec et al., 2007) was developed to assess team effectiveness on a three-point scale (0 = never or rarely; 1 = inconsistently; 2 = consistently). The scale examines behaviors related to performance in a team such as effective listening and communications, accountability to team goals, mutual dependence on the organization and each other, demonstration of decision-making ability, personal and team leadership, understanding team disadvantages and liabilities, conflict management, and innovation that provided evidence of competency. These concepts included in the scale were based on the work of Salas, Sims, and Klein (2004).

The Agency for Healthcare Research and Quality (AHRQ) has developed excellent material in a program called TeamSTEPPS® that focuses on teamwork and safety. It is a team-training curriculum designed for health care professionals that helps to improve patient safety within organizations and that provides an evidence-based teamwork system to improve communication and teamwork skills among health care professionals. TeamSTEPPS (2009) provides an instructional framework based on four team competencies—leadership, situation monitoring, mutual support, and communications. The content is presented in a multimedia format, with tools to help a health care organization plan, conduct, and evaluate its own team training program. In addition to instructor manuals and guides, there are many assessment tools focused on teamwork. The following provides a few examples of tools available in TeamSTEPPS.

The TeamSTEPPS Teamwork Perception Questionnaire (T-TPQ) is a measurement tool to help determine how an individual perceives the current state of teamwork within an organization. The TeamSTEPPS Teamwork Attitudes Questionnaire (T-TAQ) is designed to help determine whether the TeamSTEPPS tools and strategies enhanced an individual participant's attitudes toward teamwork, increased knowledge about effective team practice, and improved team skills. A TeamSTEPPS Team Assessment Questionnaire is designed to assess an individual's impressions of team behavior as it relates to patient care in her or his work setting. It includes 55 items graded on a five-point Likert scale from strongly agree to strongly disagree. The items are grouped according to the themes of team foundation, team functioning, team performance, team skills, team leadership, team climate and atmosphere, and team identity. Another tool included in TeamSTEPPS is the Team Performance Observation Tool. Using a Likert rating scale of 1 (very poor) to 5 (excellent), the observer is asked to rate a number of team attributes around the areas of team structure, leadership, situation monitoring, mutual support, and communication. In addition, there are other tools found on the TeamSTEPPS website (http:/teamstepp.AHRQ.gov/) that provide useful resources for advance practice nurses and others. It is clear from this review of these instruments and the literature in general that there is no one comprehensive instrument that addresses all of the multifactorial perspectives of teams.

To reiterate a question posed earlier in this section, what do you do when there are no instruments appropriate for the evaluation that you plan to conduct? You will need to collect that information through another source such as through the development of an evaluation protocol that asks questions about the area of interest. Even when a validated instrument is used, it becomes one component of an evaluation protocol for the collection of information.

EVALUATION OF TEAMS

With this background information in mind, how is an APN going to evaluate a team? There is no easy answer or single approach to the evaluation. However, there are a number of questions about purpose and scope of the evaluation that, once answered, will help to focus the evaluation. A number of evaluation models have been discussed in previous chapters that provide the APN with frameworks in viewing the process. There are also practical frameworks that help the APN to identify the steps and activities in evaluating a team in a concrete way. In Chapter 1, Table 1.3 outlined the basic steps in evaluation, thus setting a generic framework for evaluation. The approach described in the following, while congruent with the evaluation approach described in Chapter 1, is also concerned with the evaluation of team interactions.

Herman, Morris, and Fitz-Gibbon (1987) outline a general framework for evaluation that includes the major process categories: 1) setting the boundaries of the evaluation; 2) selecting appropriate evaluation methods; 3) collecting and analyzing information; and 4) reporting the findings. Under each major heading are a number of steps that guide the process (Table 9.4). This framework may be used to guide the process of evaluating a team by the APN. To map the evaluation process in a concise and efficient format, a logic model framework can also be used (Table 9.5). The information provided is applicable regardless if the APN is internal to an organization and asked to conduct an evaluation, or if the APN is external to the organization and is invited to conduct an evaluation.

TABLE 9.4
Practical Framework for Evaluating Health Care Teams

Activities	Focus
Set boundaries of the evaluation.	
• Determine the purposes of the evaluation.	• What are the purposes of the evaluation? Who is requesting it and how will the report be used?
• Learn all you can about the team.	
• Describe the team.	• Investigate the historical background of the team, why was it formed, has its purpose changed over time, where is it developmentally, what is the composition, to whom does it report, etc.?
• Focus the evaluation.	
• Negotiate your role.	
	• How would you succinctly describe the team?

(continued)

TABLE 9.4 (*continued*)

Activities	Focus
	• Based on the purpose, intended use, and characteristics of the team, how will you narrow the focus of the evaluation? See Table 10.2 for examples of perspectives.
	• How will you participate in the evaluation? To whom are you responsible? Will you be given access to the people and information that you need to conduct the evaluation?
Select appropriate evaluation methods.	
• Refine the description of the team.	• Why does the team exist; to whom are they responsible (broad stake-holders).
• Make sure you are asking the right questions.	
• Determine the course of action that will result from the data you supply.	• Verify and clarify what you want to address in your final report to be sure you are collecting the most appropriate data.
• Design a plan from evaluating the team.	
• Decide what to measure and observe.	• Be very clear on how the information you provide will be used so that there is a good match between purposes and col-lected information.
• Determine any associated costs with the evaluation.	
• Come to a final agreement about ser-vices and responsibilities.	• Do you have an overall plan?
	• What will you measure and observe? Have a written plan.
	• What will the evaluation cost?
	• Are you clear about your role and responsibilities?
Collect and analyze information.	
• Construct or purchase instruments.	• How will you collect the data? What resources are available to you?
• Set deadlines for data collection.	
• Determine expectations for interpreting your data.	• Do you have a written timeline for your work (e.g., Gantt chart)?
• Make sure that your data collection plan is implemented properly.	
• Analyze data with an eye on team improvement.	

(*continued*)

TABLE 9.4
Practical Framework for Evaluating Health Care Teams (*continued*)

Activities	Focus
	• Is your implementation plan complete? List all activities to be completed.
	• Address interrater reliability.
	• How can you use the data to make recommendations to enhance performance?
Report your findings.	
• Determine the format for reporting your findings.	• How will you report your findings (informal, formal, memo, email, etc.) and to whom?
• Meet with team leader and/or staff to verify factual information.	• Are your facts correct? Verify with the team leader or team members.
• Present the report.	• Leave a record of the evaluation.
• Come to closure.	• How will you come to closure with the project?

Based on Herman, J. L., Morris, L. L., & Fitz-Gibbon, C. T. (1987). *Evaluator's handbook.* Newbury Park, CA: Sage.

SETTING THE BOUNDARIES OF THE EVALUATION

In order to conduct a useful evaluation of team effectiveness, the APN must be able to set the boundaries of the evaluation so that it is a doable and useful project.

Purpose

A clear understanding of the purposes of the evaluation is imperative. This information comes from the person or persons requesting the evaluation such as a director, chief nurse or executive officer, a board, a committee, or another initiator. The purpose or purposes are varied and may include: the impact of the team on quality indicators of patient outcomes or cost savings; examination of team processes in relation to compliance with evidence-based practice guidelines and best practices; comprehensiveness of care; team group dynamics; leadership practices; and team member and patient satisfaction with care by the team. Another way to think about the evaluation is from the

TABLE 9.5
A Logic Model

Evaluation: Interdisciplinary Team on Intensive Care Unit A

Situation: Examine team effectiveness in meeting patient outcome benchmarks for length of stay (LOS) in an intensive care unit. Current data show that the LOS is 2.5 days longer than national averages. Evaluate the team to determine why the team is not meeting national benchmarks.

	Outputs		Outcomes – Impact		
Inputs	Activities	Participation	Short	Medium	Long (Impact)
Multidisciplinary team (MDs, NPs, RT, PharmD).	Conduct meeting to focus evaluation.	Leadership	Awareness of barriers.	Leadership satisfied with changes.	High performance multidisciplinary team.
Time devoted for rounds.	Meet to discuss work processes of patient management to move patients across continuum of care.	Leadership of multidisciplinary team.	Removal of barriers.	Improved function of multidisciplinary team.	Increased esteem of multidisciplinary team.
Combined EMR and paper for writing orders and progress notes).		Members of each discipline in team.	Education of multidisciplinary team	Average LOS met or LOS less than national average.	Increased satisfaction of team members, staff, and patients/families.
Leadership who wants improved outcomes.	Observe conduct of rounds, flow of information, and interactions.	Multidisciplinary team.	New attitudes and awareness.	Integration of EBPs and best practices.	
Strong organizational commitment to evidence-based practice (EBP) with resource support.	Meetings to discuss flow.	Nursing staff and support staff (transcriber of orders, other departments).	Knowledge about EBP and best practices.	Policies, procedures, and protocols followed.	Sustained cost savings from shorter LOS.
Data on LOS.	Observe work patterns related to transfer/ discharge.	Nursing staff.	Revision of process maps for transfer and discharge.	Better communications.	Better overall patient outcomes.
Available national data for similar academic medical centers.	Review protocols for admission and discharge from unit.	Written policies, procedures, and protocols.	Facilitator to help improve group communications, trust, mutual respect, and common goals.	Cost savings from shorter LOS.	
			Revision of policies, procedures, and protocols.		

Assumptions: High functioning multidisciplinary teams can provide comprehensive care. LOS can be facilitated by input of all team members using protocols based on EBP to move patients in a timely manner from one level of care to the next.

External Factors: Reimbursement for care is tied to LOS; longer than aveage LOS are not reimburse by some insurers and create a huge burden on the health care facility to absorb those costs. EBPs can decrease LOS, if followed.

perspective of problems. What are the specific problems with the team that are to be addressed? This approach also helps to identify desired outcomes from the evaluation and sets the evaluation criteria to be used. Because evaluation information is used for decision making, it is helpful to know who is going to receive the information and for what purpose the information will be used (e.g., team redesign, continued funding of the team, improvement in patient outcomes). All of this information helps to shape the evaluation process.

Gaining Knowledge About the Team and Describing the Team

The APN may or may not have knowledge of the team and should take the time to conduct a comprehensive assessment of the team. Even if the APN thinks he or she knows the team, the APN must take a fresh unbiased look at the team from the eyes of an evaluator. Examples of areas to consider are: historical background of the team (e.g., When was it formed? For what purpose? Who started the team?); the setting in which the team functions and how it is tied to the organizational structure; changes in the purpose of the team over time; the membership of the team; the time each member has been on the team; the team's organization; the team leaders; how work gets done; and where the team is developmentally. This information can be gathered through discussions, observation, and review of written materials. Once necessary information has been collected, the APN will be able to describe the team and categorize it according to type, developmental level, work patterns and processes, and outcomes.

Focusing the Evaluation and Negotiating the Evaluator Role

Once the APN has collected the information and formulated a description of the team, the APN can begin to clarify the rationale and objectives for the evaluation and narrow the scope. This should lead to a brief outline of purpose, rationale, objectives, and scope, which should be shared with the person or persons requesting the evaluation to verify and clarify a common view of the focus of the evaluation. This is also a time to negotiate the evaluator role. Be clear about the expectations, responsibilities, deliverables, timeline, and the person to whom the APN will report findings. The APN should verify access to information and people for the conduct of the work, and determine what the team members have been told about the evaluation and who provided that information. In addition, the APN must identify the contact person who will act as facilitator if issues occur in the conduct of the evaluation. The APN should discuss what format the final report should take and who should receive it. Finally, the conditions under which the work will be done should be addressed. If the APN is an outside consultant, conditions of work and compensation is addressed through a contract. If the APN is internal to the organization, how will this work be calculated into his/her current workload?

Is there anyone available to help or provide support for data gathering? These and other questions need to be addressed prospectively to avoid misunderstandings later.

SELECTING APPROPRIATE EVALUATION METHODS

To move the evaluation process forward, a number of refinements, double checks, and design and measurement decisions need to be made.

Refine Description of the Team and Re-examine the Approach

In selecting appropriate evaluation methods, the APN should further refine and double check the description of the team, the rationale for the team, and the goals/objectives of the evaluation. This may seem like redundancy, but as the APN continues to work and plan, there may be new information and subtle changes in direction that influence the approach including what questions and observations need to be completed in order to get to the heart of the evaluation. The APN will also want to be clear on the outcomes on which to focus (e.g., processes, outcomes). The APN should have a very clear understanding of how the resultant information will be used so that there is a good match between purposes and collected information.

Design a Plan Including Measurement

The next step is to develop a detailed, step-by-step written plan of activities, data to be collected, methods of collection, timeline for collection, and sources of data. Knowledge of the organization/system and team will help the APN make these determinations. The APN should decide what to measure and observe, and may wish to measure contextual characteristics, participant characteristics, processes, patient outcomes, or costs. The variables that the APN decides to investigate must be operationally defined to determine how they can best be measured. For example, to investigate team communication patterns, the APN first must define communication patterns. The definition might include verbal interactions among team members, verbal interactions of team members with bedside staff nurses, written documentation of plan of care, or exchange of information at team conferences. How the concept is operationalized will drive options for measurement. For example, the definition given earlier regarding verbal interactions among team members could be investigated by observation of team members at work, by a questionnaire, or both. The evaluator must decide what method or methods of measurement are available and which will best meet the objectives of the evaluation. If there is any cost associated with measurement such as purchase of instruments, these costs need to be included in a budget for approval by the sponsor of the evaluation.

The APN must recognize the state of the science of evaluation of teams. Interpretive difficulties arise when examining how team outcomes are conceptualized and measured. Like the construct team, the outcome is also multi-dimensional, and poorly conceptualized outcomes make comparisons across studies difficult. Team studies usually examine processes or outcomes of teams, but not the linkages between the two (Schmitt et al., 1988; Schofield & Amodeo, 1999). Understanding the state of the science in evaluation of health teams will help to maintain realistic expectations of what can be accomplished from an evaluation.

Collecting and Analyzing Information

In this phase the APN constructs or purchases instruments, creates an evaluation protocol, and sets timelines for data collection and for analyzing the data with an eye on team improvement, which will be communicated in the form of summary remarks, conclusions, and recommendations.

Construct or Purchase Data Collection Instruments

Depending upon the purposes and objectives of the evaluation, the APN will either create her or his own data collection instrument, purchase validated instruments, or use a combination of both. If any instruments are purchased, be sure that the intended purpose of the instrument and the purpose of the evaluation are congruent. For example, the Collaboration Assessment Tool (Baggs et al., 1992, 1997) was designed to measure nurse-physician collaboration in making specific decisions about patient care; it will not be useful to provide a comprehensive view of a team's overall effectiveness. Another instrument such as TeamSTEPPS Team Assessment Questionnaire is better suited to provide a comprehensive view. Regardless if the instruments are evaluator created or purchased, the APN must follow a timeline for data collection. If another person is assisting with data collection, the APN will need to orient that person to the instrument and data collection process to ensure interrater reliability.

Data Analysis

Once data are collected and organized in a usable format, the data analysis is conducted. Quantitative data may be entered into a spread sheet of statistical analysis program such as Statistical Package for Social Sciences (SPSS). Qualitative data may be examined using content analysis or other qualitative data analysis methods. The data analyzed should be related clearly to the objectives outlined for the evaluation. As the APN analyzes the data, he/she must keep an eye on opportunities for quality improvement of team effectiveness around the areas evaluated. Are there any national standards or benchmarks that may be useful to frame the data collected? The APN should think about recommendations that may assist the decision makers who will receive the report.

REPORTING THE FINDINGS

Once data analysis is completed and findings formulated, the APN may wish to meet with the team leader and/or team members to discuss and follow up on the findings if this has been approved by the initiator of the evaluation. Such a meeting is directed at transparency and provides the opportunity to correct any factual information that was incorrect.

The next step is preparing the final report. The format of the report is something that is negotiated during an earlier step in the process. The report can be informal or formal. An informal report may take the form of an e-mail or a memo; a formal report may require a detailed written report with an executive summary. A formal report may also include a presentation to a board or a committee with a detail review of the processes and outcomes of the evaluation project. Regardless if the report is informal or formal, the APN should provide a tangible record of the evaluation in the form of a written report or electronic file, and a copy for his/her records.

The question of communicating the results of the evaluation with the team that was evaluated needs to be addressed. That decision usually lies in the hands of the person or persons who requested the evaluation. That person or persons must decide what information they wish to share with the team and how the information will be communicated.

Come to closure with the person or persons who requested the evaluation, those who assisted with the conduct of the evaluation, and the participants in the evaluation. It is clear from the brief overview of the conduct of an evaluation that it is a complex process that requires many decisions to be made along the way by the evaluator. That is true if conducting an informal focused evaluation of a team or a formal comprehensive evaluation. The principles are the same regardless of approach and should lead to useful information for the decision makers.

SUMMARY

This chapter proposed to provide an overview of the state of the science of teams in health care and what is known about their effectiveness. Through a review of the literature, a view of the complexity of health care and teams delivering care was presented. The recently published core competencies for interprofessional collaborative practice were briefly discussed, and the domains and specific competencies outlined from the report. A list of variables that have been used in evaluating teams was offered. It was made clear that there are theoretical/conceptual and methodological challenges in the evaluation of teams that prevent a clear link between processes and outcomes. However, from a practical perspective, teams still need to be evaluated. To assist with this process a generic approach to evaluation of a team was discussed. In addition, a logic model was presented to provide a concise view of the overall process. Further development in team theory and methodology will move the understanding of how teams contribute to health care outcomes with the precision and clarity desired.

REFERENCES

Agency for Healthcare Research and Quality. TeamSTEPPS. Washington, DC: Author, U.S. Department of Health and Human Services. Retrieved from http://teamstepps.ahrq.gov/ (Accessed January 2012).

Aiken, L., Clarke, S., Cheung, R., Sloane, D., & Silber, J. (2004). Relationship between patient mortality and nurses' level of education. *Journal of the American Medical Association, 291*(11), 1322–1323.

Aiken, L., Clarke, S., & Sloane, D. (2002). Hospital staffing, organizational and quality of care cross-national findings. *International Journal for Quality in Healthcare, 14*(1), 5–13.

Andretta, P. B. (2010). A typology for health care teams. *Health Care Management Review, 35*(4), 345–354.

Ash, L., & Miller, C. (2010). Interprofessional collaboration for improving patient and population health. In M. E. Zaccagnini & K. W. White (Eds.), *The doctor of nursing practice essentials: A model for advanced practice nursing* (pp. 235–272). Boston, MA: Jones and Bartlett Publishers.

Baggs, J. G., Ryan, S. A., Phelps, C. E., Richeson, J. F., & Johnson, J. E. (1992). The association between interdisciplinary collaboration and patient outcomes in a medical intensive care unit. *Heart & Lung, 21*(1), 18–24.

Baggs, J. G., & Schmitt, M. H. (1988). Collaboration between nurses and physicians. *Image: Journal of Nursing Scholarship, 20*, 145–149.

Baggs, J. G., & Schmitt, M. H. (1997). Nurses' and resident physicians' perception of the process of collaboration in a MICU. *Research in Nursing & Health, 20*, 71–80.

Baggs, J. G., Schmitt, M. H., Mushlin, A. I., Eldredge, D. H., Oakes, D., & Hutson, A. D. (1997). Nurse-physician collaboration and satisfaction with the decision making process in critical care units. *American Journal of Critical Care, 6*(5), 393–399.

Baggs, J. G., Schmitt, M. H., Mushlin, A. I., Mitchell, P. H., Eldredge, D. H., Oakes, D., & Hutson, A. D. (1999). Association between nurse-physician collaboration and patient outcomes in three intensive care units. *Critical Care Medicine, 27*(90), 1991–1998.

Boaro, N., Fancott, C., Baker, R., Velji, K., & Andreoli, A. (2010). Using SBAR to improve communication in interprofessional rehabilitation teams. *Journal of Interprofessional Care, 24*(1), 111–114.

Boult, C., Green, A. F., Boult, L. B., Pacala, J. T., Synder, C., & Leff, B. (2009). Successful models of comprehensive care for older adults with chronic conditions: Evidence for the Institute of Medicine's "retooling for an aging American" report. *Journal of American Geriatric Society, 57*(12), 2328–2337.

Boyle, D. K., & Kochinda, C. (2004). Enhancing collaborative communication of nurse and physician leadership in two intensive care units. *Journal of Nursing Administration, 34*(2), 60–70.

Bronstein, L. R. (2002). Index of interdisciplinary collaboration. *Social Work Research, 26*(2), 113–123.

Choi, B. C. K., & Pak, A. W. P. (2006). Multidisciplinarity, interdisciplinarity, and transdisciplinarity in health research, services, education and policy: 1. Definitions, objectives, and evidence of effectiveness. *Clinical Investigation Medicine, 29*(6), 351–364.

Cowan, M. J., Shapiro, M., Hays, R. D., Afifi, A., Vazirani, S., Ward, C. R., & Ettner, S. L. (2006). The effect of a multidisciplinary hospitalist/physician and advanced practice nurse collaboration on hospital costs. *Journal of Nursing Administration, 36*(2), 79–85.

DeChairo-Marino, A. E., Jordon-Marsh, M., Traiger, G., & Saulo, M. (2001). Nurse/physician collaboration: Action research and the lessons learned. *Journal of Nursing Administration, 31*(5), 223–232.

Durbin, C. G. (2006). Team model: Advocating for the optimal method of care delivery in the intensive care unit. *Critical Care Medicine, 34*(Suppl. 3), S12–S17.

Famadas, J. C., Frick, K. D., Haydar, Z. R., Nicewander, D., Ballard, D., & Boult, C. (2008). The effects of interdisciplinary outpatient geriatrics on the use, costs, and quality of health services in the fee-for-service environment. *Aging Clinical Experimental Research, 20*(6), 556–561.

Farrell, M. P., Heinemann G, D., & Schmitt, M. H. (1986). Informed roles, rituals and humor in interdisciplinary health teams: Their relation to stages of group development. *International Journal of Small Group Research, 2*(2), 143–162.

Farrell, M. P., Heinemann, G. D., & Schmitt, M. H. (1988). Informal roles, rituals, and humor in interdisciplinary health care teams: Their relation to stages of group development. *International Journal of Small Group Research, 2*(2), 143–162.

Farrell, M. P., Schmitt, M. H., & Heinemann, G. D. (1988). Organizational environments of interdisciplinary health care teams: Impact on team development and implications for consultation. *International Journal of Small Group Research, 4*(1), 31–54.

Farrell, M. P., Schmitt, M. H., & Heinemann, G. D. (2001). Informal roles and the stages of interdisciplinary team development. *Journal of Interprofessional Care, 15*, 281–293.

Feiger, S. M., & Schmitt, M. H. (1979). Collegiality in interdisciplinary health teams: Its measurement and its effects. *Social Science & Medicine, 13A*, 217–229.

Freshman, B., Rubino, L., & Chassiakos, Y. R. (2010). *Collaboration across the disciplines in health care.* Sudbury, MA: Jones and Bartlett Publishers.

Friese, C., Lake, E., Aiken, L., Silver, J., & Sochalski, J. (2008). Hospital nurse practice environments and outcomes for surgical oncology patients. *Health Services Research, 43*(4), 1145–1163.

Grumbach, K., & Bodenheimer, T. (2004). Can health care teams improve primary care practice? *Journal of the American Medical Association, 291*(10), 1246–1251.

Halstead, L. S. (1976). Team care in chronic illness: A critical review of the literature of the past 25 years. *Archives of Physical Medicine and Rehabilitation, 57*, 507–511.

Heintz, C., & Origgi, G. (2005). Rethinking interdisciplinary: Emergent issues. Interdisciplines. Retrieved from http://www.interdisciplines.org/interdisciplinarity/papers/11

Herman, J. L., Morris, L. L., & Fitz-Gibbon, C. T. (1987). *Evaluator's handbook.* Newbury Park, CA: Sage.

Horbar, J., Plsek, P., Leahy, K., & Ford, P. (2004). The Vermont Oxford network: Improving quality and safety through multidisciplinary collaboration. *NeoReviews, 5*(2), e42–e49.

Houldin, A. D., Naylor, M. D., & Haller, D. G. (2004). Physician-nurse collaboration in research in the 21st century. *Journal of Clinical Oncology, 22*(5), 774–776.

Ingersoll, G. L., & Schmitt, M. (2004). Interdisciplinary collaboration, team functioning, and patient safety. In Institute of Medicine, *Keeping patient safe: Transforming the work environment of nurses* (pp. 341–383). Washington, DC: National Academies Press.

Institute of Medicine. (2003). *Health professions education: A bridge to quality.* Washington, DC: National Academies Press.

Institute of Medicine. (2010). *The future of nursing: Leading change, advancing health.* Washington, DC: The National Academies Press.

Institute of Medicine Roundtable on Evidence-Based Medicine. (2008). *Learning healthcare system concepts.* Washington, DC: The National Academies Press.

Interprofessional Education Collaborative Expert Panel. (2011). *Core competencies for interprofessional collaborative practice: Report of an expert panel.* Washington, DC: Author.

Janis, I. L. (1982). *Groupthink* (2nd ed.). Boston, MA: Houghton Mifflin.

Kim, M. M., Barnato, A. E., Angus, D. C., Fleisher, L. A., & Kahn, J. M. (2010). The effect of multidisciplinary care teams on intensive care unit mortality. *Archives of Internal Medicine, 170*(4), 369–376.

Klimoski, R. J., & Mohammed, S. (1994). Team mental model: Construct or metaphor? *Journal of Management, 20,* 403–437.

Knaus, W. A., Draper, E. A., Wagner, D. P., & Zimmerman, J. E. (1986). An evaluation of outcome from intensive care in major medical centers. *Annals of Internal Medicine, 104*(3), 410–418.

Korner, M. (2010). Interprofessional teamwork in medical rehabilitation: A comparison of multidisciplinary and interdisciplinary team approach. *Clinical Rehabilitation, 24*(8), 745–755.

Kozlowski, S. W. J., & Ilgen, D. R. (2006). Enhancing the effectiveness of work groups and teams. *Psychological Science in Public Interest, 7*(3), 77–124.

Leathard, A. (Ed.), (1994). *Going interprofessional: Working together for health and welfare.* London: Routledge.

Lemieux-Charles, L., & McGuire, W. L. (2006). What do we know about health care team effectiveness? A review of the literature. *Medical Care Research and Review, 63*(3), 263–300.

Lorimer, W., & Manion, J. (1996, Spring). Team-based organizations: Leading the essential transformation. *PFCA Review, 15,* 9.

Malec, J. F., Torsher, L. C., Dunn, W. F., Wiegmann, D. A., Arnold, J. J., Brown, D. A., & Phatak, V. (2007). The Mayo high performance teamwork scale: Reliability and validity for evaluating key crew resource management skills. *Simulation Healthcare, 2*(1), 4–10.

Marks, M. A., Mathieu, J. E., & Zaccaro, S. J. (2001). A temporally based framework and taxonomy of team processes. *Academy of Management Review, 26,* 356–376.

Massachusetts Institute of Technology. (2011). *The third revolution: The convergence of the life sciences, physical sciences, and engineering.* Washington, DC: Author.

McClure, M. L., Poulin, M. A., Sovie, M. D., & Wandelt, M. A. (1983). *Magnet hospitals: Attraction and retention of professional nurses.* Kansas City, MO: American Academy of Nursing.

Meier, D. E., & Beresford, L. (2010). Palliative care in long-term care: How can hospital teams interface? *Journal of Palliative Care, 13*(2), 556–561.

Mills, P., Neily, J., & Dunn, E. (2008). Teamwork and communication in surgical teams: Implications for patient safety. *Journal of American College of Surgeons, 206*(1), 107–112.

Mitchell, P. H., Shannon, S. E., Cain, K. C., & Hegyvary, S. T. (1996). Critical care outcomes: Linking structures, processes, and organizational and clinical outcomes. *American Journal of Critical Care, 5*, 353–363.

Nelson, E. C., Batalden, P. B., & Godfrey, M. M. (2007). *Quality by design: A clinical microsystems approach*. San Francisco, CA: Jossey-Bass.

Nelson, E. C., Batalden, P. B., Huber, T. P., Mohr, J. J., Godfrey, M. M., Headrick, L. A., & Wasson, J. H. (2002). Microsystems in health care: Part 1. Learning from high-performing front-line clinical units. *Joint Commission Journal on Quality Improvement, 25*, 654–668.

Neumann, V., Gutenbrunner, C., Fialda-Moser, V., Christodoulou, N., Varela, E., Giustine, A., & Delarque, A. (2010). Interdisciplinary team working in physical and rehabilitation medicine. *Journal of Rehabilitation Medicine, 42*(1), 4–8.

Paulus, P. B., & Nijstad, B. A. (Eds.), (2003). *Group creativity: Innovation through collaboration*. New York: Oxford University Press.

Pezzin, L. E., Feldman, P. H., Mongoven, J. M., McDonald, M. V., Gerber, L. M., & Peng, T. R. (2011). *Journal of General Internal Medicine, 26*(3), 280–286.

Pisano, G. P., & Verganti, R. (2008). Which kind of collaboration is right for you? *Harvard Business Review, 86*(12), 78–86.

Pronovost, P. J., Berenholtz, S. M., Goeschel, C., Needman, D., Hyzy, R., Welsh, R., ... Sexton, J. B. (2008). Improving patient safety in intensive care units in Michigan. *Journal of Critical Care, 23*(2), 207–221.

Pyne, J. M., Fortney, J. C., Curran, G. M., Tripathi, S., Atkinson, J. H., Kilbourne, A. M., ... Gifford, A. L. (2011). Effectiveness of collaborative care for depression in human immunodeficiency virus clinics. *Archives of Internal Medicine, 171*(1), 23–31.

Reader, T. W., Fin, R., Mearns, K., & Cuthbertson, B. (2009). Developing a team performance framework for the intensive care unit. *Critical Care Medicine, 37*(5), 1787–1793.

Reid-Ponte, P., Creta, A., & Joy, C. (2011). Exemplary professional practice. In K. Drenkard, G. Wolf, & S. H. Morgan (Eds.), *Magnet: The next generation –Nurses making a difference* (pp. 68–69). Silver Spring, MD: American Nurses Credentialing Center.

Rocco, N., Scher, K., Basberg, B., Yalamanchi, S., & Baker-Genaw, K. (2011). Patient-centered plan-of-care tool for improving clinical outcomes. *Quality Management in Health Care, 20*(2), 89–97.

Salas, E., Sims, D. E., & Klein, C. (2004). Cooperation and teamwork at work. In C. D. Spielberger (Ed.), *Encyclopedia of applied psychology* (Vol. 1, pp. 497–505). San Diego, CA: Academic Press.

Sassou, K., & Reason, J. (1999). Team errors: Definition and taxonomy. *Reliability Engineering and Systems Safety, 65*, 1–9.

Schmitt, M. H. (2001). Collaboration improves the quality of care: Methodological challenges and evidence from U.S. health care research. *Journal of Interprofessional Care, 15*, 47–66.

Schmitt, M. H., Farrell, M. P., & Heinemann, G. D. (1988). Conceptual and methodological problems in studying the effects of interdisciplinary teams. *The Gerontologist, 40*, 343.

Schofield, R. F., & Amodeo, M. (1999). Interdisciplinary teams in health care and humans services settings: Are they effective? *Health & Social Work, 24*, 210–219.

Senge, P. M. (1990). *The fifth discipline.* New York: Doubleday Currency.

Shortell, S. M., Zimmerman, J. E., Gillies, R. R., Duffy, J., Devers, K., Rousseau, D. M., & Knaus, W. A. (1992). Continuously improving patient care: Practical lessons and an assessment tool from the national ICU study. *Quality Review Bulletin, 18*(5), 150–155.

Shortell, S. M., Zimmerman, J. E., Rousseau, D. M., Gillies, R. R., Wagner, D. P., Draper, E. A., ... Duffy, J. (1994). The performance of intensive care units: Does good management make a difference? *Medical Care, 32,* 508–525.

Singh, J., & Fleming, L. (2010). Lone inventors as sources of breakthroughs: Myth or reality? *Management Science, 56*(1), 41–56.

Smith, M. K. (2005). Bruce W. Tuckman – Forming, storming, norming and performing in group. *The Encyclopaedia of Informal Education.* Retrieved from www.infed.org/thinkers/tuckman.htm

Sorrells-Jones, J. (1997). The challenge of making it real: Interdisciplinary practice in a "seamless" organization. *Nursing Administration Quarterly, 21*(2), 20–30.

TeamSTEPPS. (2009). *Team strategies and tools to enhance performance and patient safety.* Rockville, MD: Agency for Healthcare Research and Quality, U. S. Department of Health and Human Services.

Tuckman, B. W. (1965). Development sequence of small groups. *Psychological Bulletin, 63,* 384–399.

Tuckman, B. W., & Jensen, M. A. (1977). Stages of small group development revisited. *Group and Organizational Studies, 2,* 419–427.

Upenieks, V. V., Lee, E. A., Flanagan, M. E., & Doebbeling, B. N. (2009). Healthcare Team Vitality Instrument (HTVI): Developing a tool assessing healthcare team functioning. *Journal of Advanced Nursing, 66*(1), 168–176.

Vrije University Amsterdam. Retrieved from http://www.bio.vu.nl/vakgroepen/bens/HTML/transdisciplinair.html

Weick, K. E., & Roberts, K. H. (1993). Collective mind in organizations: Heedful interrelating on flight decks. *Administrative Science Quarterly, 38,* 357–381.

Wiecha, J., & Pollard, T. (2004). The interdisciplinary eHealth Team: Chronic care for the future. *Journal of Medical Internet Research, 6,* e22. Retrieved from http://www.jmir.org/2004/3/e22

Wuchty, S. B., Jones, F., & Uzzi, B. (2007). The increasing dominance of teams in production of knowledge. *Science, 316*(5827), 1036–1039.

Xyrichis, A., & Ream, E. (2008). Teamwork: A concept analysis. *Journal of Advanced Nursing, 61*(2), 232–241.

Zwarenstein, M. J., Goldman, M. J., & Reeves, S. (2009). Interprofessional collaboration: Effects of practice-based interventions on professional practice and healthcare outcomes. *Cochrane Database of Systematic Reviews,* (3), CD000072.

TEN

Translating Outcomes From Evaluation to Health Policy

Deanna E. Grimes, Richard M. Grimes,
and Christine A. Brosnan

"Knowing is not enough; we must apply. Willing is not enough; we must do."

Goethe

INTRODUCTION

APNs may question the relevance of health policy to their patients' needs and to their ability to take care of their patients. One might also wonder why the American Association of Colleges of Nursing (AACN) specified Health Care Policy for Advocacy in Health Care as one of the *Essentials for Doctoral Education for Advanced Nursing Practice* (AACN, 2006) and one of the *Essentials of Master's Education in Nursing* (AACN, 2011). The purpose of this chapter is to address why and how APNs can influence health policy. This chapter will: 1) define health policy; 2) address the question of why nurses are involved in health policy; 3) outline guidelines for analyzing a health policy; 4) summarize the policy process; 5) describe how nurses can influence health policy with outcome evaluation; and 6) describe the nursing roles of advocacy and leadership in the policy arena. A case study and questions are provided to enable the reader to apply the principles of this chapter.

WHAT IS HEALTH POLICY?

There are almost as many definitions of health policy as there are policies. A general definition of policy is the "authoritative guidelines that direct human behavior toward specific goals, in either the private or the public sector" (Hanley, 2002). Nurses are familiar with the myriad of policies within the private sector, such as organizational policies in the workplace dealing with staffing, chain of command, vacation time, evaluation, and salary. Nurses also live with countless public sector policies, such as the laws that determine licensure requirements, taxes, building codes, disposal of wastes, speed limits, and driving regulations. Some policy experts define policy only in terms of the public sector. Longest (2006, p. 7) defines policy as "authoritative decisions made in the legislative, executive, or judicial branches of government that are intended to direct or influence the actions, behaviors, or decisions of others." The term *authoritative* is key to most definitions of policy and suggests that there is a legal or administrative power or command behind the policy. When policies influence health, the determinants of health, or the use of the health care system, they can then be called health policies. Health policies can impact entire populations as well as selected individuals in the population. The authors of this chapter recognize that private sector as well as public sector policies influence health. As an example, hospital policies that control the quality and numbers of nurses on any shift can contribute to the health of patients as well as the health of the nursing staff.

The list of what constitutes a health policy can be extremely long and varied. The list covers issues at the national level, such as health care reform, insurance for the currently uninsured, Medicare prescription drug policies, and policies regulating over-the-counter drugs and diet supplements. State health policies range from Medicaid policies to who is licensed to practice as an APN. Because states have the ultimate authority for the public's health and well-being, state policy also covers issues such as sanitation, the safety of the water supply, speed limits on the highways, and immunizations required to attend school, all of which impact health.

WHY ARE NURSES INVOLVED IN HEALTH POLICY?

According to the AACN's *Essentials of Doctoral Education for Advanced Nursing Practice*, Health Care Policy for Advocacy in Health Care is Essential V (2006). The AACN (2006, p. 14) further specifies the expectations of the graduate of a DNP program with respect to policy and advocacy as follows:

1. Critically analyze health policy proposals, health polices, and related issues from the perspective of consumers, nursing, other health professions, and other stakeholders in policy and public forums.
2. Demonstrate leadership in the development and implementation of institutional, local, state, federal, and/or international health policy.

3. Influence policy makers through active participation on committees, boards, or task forces at the institutional, local, state, regional, national, and/or international levels to improve health care delivery and outcomes.

4. Educate others, including policy makers at all levels, regarding nursing, health policy, and patient care outcomes.

5. Advocate for the nursing profession within the policy and health care communities.

6. Develop, evaluate, and provide leadership for health care policy that shapes health care financing, regulation and delivery.

7. Advocate for social justice, equity, and ethical policies within all health care arenas.

Thus, one of the reasons APNs are involved in health policy is that involvement is an expectation of the APN role. Another equally important reason is that health policy has a downward influence on everything that happens and everything done in the health care system, including all aspects of nursing practice. Perhaps the most comprehensive depiction of the totality of the influence of health policy on health and health care can be seen in Figure 10.1 (Aday, Begley, Lairson, & Balkrishnan, 2004).

The model was discussed in Chapter 3 as a framework for evaluation. It is provided here because of its relevance to the influences of health policy. A quick review of definitions in the model in Figure 10.1: 1) Structure refers to the composition of the health care system, the populations it serves, and the environment in which the system exists; 2) process is what providers do in the system and the health states of those who seek help from the system; and 3) outcomes are what the system is trying to achieve. The criteria are the standards whereby one can evaluate the outcomes from both a clinical or patient perspective and from a population perspective. One can expand the content in each of the boxes in the model to reflect the reality of one's nursing practice. For example, an APN providing primary care in a public health clinic in a Medically Underserved Community (MUC) has different available resources than one providing primary care in a private hospital outpatient clinic in a medical center. Additionally, patient needs are different in the different types of settings, and not all patients or communities achieve the same outcomes from their encounter with health care. Some are sicker at the onset or do not have the resources to follow a treatment or prevention plan. And some never get to receive the primary care they need. This model is used as a reminder that health policy, whether federal, state or local, impacts every aspect of the health care system and the health of the population served.

Nurses can monitor the impact of health policy on patient and population outcomes. And, even more importantly, nurses can use that information to influence change in health policy. More on this later in this chapter.

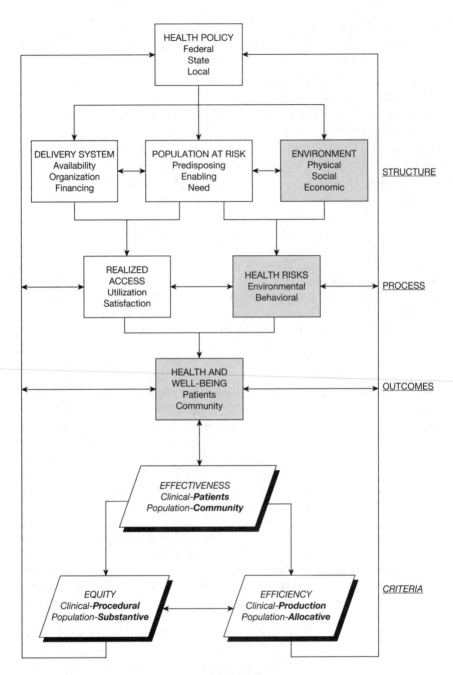

FIGURE 10.1
Framework for applying health services research in evaluating health policy.
Adapted with permission from *Evaluating the health care system* by L. A. Aday,
C. E. Begley, D. R. Lairson, and R. Balkrishnan, 2004,
Chicago: Health Administration Press, p. 14.

GUIDELINES FOR ANALYZING A HEALTH POLICY

In order to use health policy to benefit patients, communities, and the nursing profession, and to influence the development of new policy or change in existing health policy, it is useful to have a framework for understanding policies and the policy process. The policy process, according to Block (2008), is simply a way to solve problems. One may be trying to understand a new health policy in order to implement it or to analyze an existing health policy in order to change it. Policy analysis is the systematic study or appraisal of existing or proposed policies according to their background, purpose, content, and anticipated or actual effects (Hanley, 2002). The framework for policy analysis described by Stokey and Zeckhauser (1978) is a useful approach because it begins with the problem that the policy purports to solve. The five steps of their problem-focused analysis are: 1) establishing the context; 2) laying out the alternatives; 3) predicting the consequences; 4) valuing the outcomes; and 5) making a choice. These steps are amplified here with questions to address for each step.

1. Establishing the context requires one to assess the circumstances surrounding the policy. One might ask some of the following questions: What is the underlying problem that the policy addresses and how is the problem defined? What are the background factors (e.g., history, emerging science, social, political, legal, ethical, economics) leading to the problem? For example, the problem underlying the addition of Medicare drug coverage was defined by some as the high cost of drugs and by others as the inability of the elderly to pay for their drugs. The difference is subtle but real and leads to different solutions. If the costs of drugs are too high, then one would establish a policy to control costs. If elderly Americans do not have money for their drugs, then one would develop a policy to pay for the drugs. Another set of questions relating to the context focus on the major players in the environment. Who (e.g., governmental agency, community group, private enterprise, etc.) is defining the problem? Who are the stakeholders in this policy; i.e., who has something to gain or lose from the policy? The stakeholders may or may not have power, but they can and do have influence. Note that the focus is not just about the "political context" but rather about the entire environment surrounding a problem. Another important question might relate to the objectives of the policy; i.e., what were the intended outcomes from the policy?
2. Laying out the alternatives relies on knowing how the problem was defined, as described in the preceding. Each definition of the problem may lead to alternative courses of action. And each stakeholder may have a different perspective on the "correct" course of action. Those who desire to influence the policy alternatives must provide additional information to expand the understanding of and available choices for different courses of action.

3. Predicting the consequences of the alternative actions also relies on an understanding of how the problem was defined. The consequences of lowering the costs of drugs are certainly different from covering the costs of drugs with expanded insurance. One could explore different analytic approaches to predict the consequences, e.g., economic versus efficacy, and the likelihood of each consequence.
4. Valuing the outcomes suggests that not everyone will view the outcomes of a policy through the same lens. Policy outcomes often are evaluated according to criteria similar to those used to define the problem (e.g., values of equity or justice, emphasis on liberty for the individual versus safety for society, ethical beliefs, economics, benefits to whom).
5. Evaluate whether the outcomes achieved or desired are the preferred outcomes. What is/was the preferred course of action? From which perspective? What can one conclude about the efficacy of the existent policy?

THE POLICY PROCESS (FIGURE 10.2)

Among the many published explanatory models of the public policy process, the one published by Longest (2006) stands out for its comprehensiveness and application for nursing. Longest describes three major phases, all of which can be impacted by nursing. The phases are policy formulation, policy implementation, and policy modification. The *policy formulation phase* is characterized by two separate sets of activities: *agenda setting* and *development of legislation*. If there is formal enactment of legislation, then one moves to *policy implementation*, which is composed of activities dealing with *rulemaking* and *operations*. Once a policy is put into operation, there is opportunity for a feedback loop to a *policy modification phase* where individuals, organizations, and governmental agencies can influence new phases of *policy formulation* and *policy implementation*.

Most of the information on the phases of the policy process is self-explanatory, however, the activities of *agenda setting* deserve further clarification and amplification, the reason being that this is the time in health policy formulation where nursing experience, expertise, and information from program evaluation are needed most. According to Longest (2006), agenda setting is comprised of problems, possible solutions, and political circumstances. When these conditions coalesce around an issue, a window of opportunity for change opens. This part of the model is based on the 1995 work of Kingdon, who conceptualized three streams of activities (e.g., a problem stream, a policy stream, and a political stream), all equally important. The *problem stream* defines the problem; the *policy stream* defines the policy goals of the stakeholders; and the *political stream* describes the political environment and power at the time (Hanley, 2002). Much of the

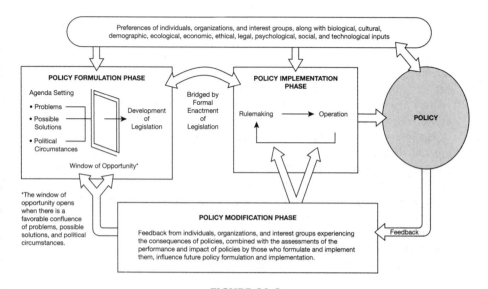

FIGURE 10.2
A Model of the Public Policymaking Process in the United States.
From Longest, B. B. (2006). *Health policymaking in the United States* (4th Ed.).
Chicago, IL: Health Administration Press.

content discussed in the previous section on policy analysis is relevant to agenda setting. The major questions are: What is the problem and how is it defined? How are various stakeholders defining the problem? What is the social, ethical, scientific, etc., background of the problem? Who are the stakeholders in the context of the problem under question? What outcomes are desired by the stakeholders? Which alternative solutions are available and desired by the various stakeholders?

INFLUENCING HEALTH POLICY WITH OUTCOME EVALUATION

Sometimes the window of opportunity to provide good information to policy makers is very narrow and, at other times, the window is partially open for long periods of time. An example of a narrow window was the time following the terrorist attack on the United States on September 11, 2001, also known as 9-11. Health care professionals and organizations defined the problem as lack of education and training for disasters, particularly bioterrorism, for health care providers. The federal government defined the problem in terms of lack of preparedness and made grant money available for education and training of health professionals. Some state boards of nursing defined the problem similarly and determined that continuing education in bioterrorism should be a requirement for nursing licensure. In the year following 9-11, those who already had the knowledge or experience in preventing infectious diseases were poised to receive funding to provide the training. Many nurses fit into that category.

Contrast that situation with that of the wide window around the HIV screening policies in the case study in this chapter (Box 10.1). The window for changing the policies has been partially open since 1987. During the ensuing years, nurses have adapted their practices to implement the changing policies in general outpatient clinics, prenatal clinics, public health clinics, delivery rooms, emergency departments, HIV treatment centers, and schools of nursing. One hopes that nurses are evaluating and publishing outcomes for their patients and the populations they serve as the new screening procedures are implemented. Publishing or disseminating such information in other ways helps to establish one's expertise in order to be able to influence future HIV screening and treatment policies. Because nurses are required to implement screening policies, nurses also should be serving on the government panels that devise the guidelines and on the committees within the health care organizations required to implement the guidelines.

ADVOCACY AND LEADERSHIP IN HEALTH POLICY

Nursing has a tradition of advocating for health policies that benefit patients. Florence Nightingale campaigned for effective care of hospitalized patients. Lillian Wald struggled to give poor women and children equal access to health care. Margaret Sanger fought to provide women with a choice about childbearing. These and many other nurses understood the connection between health policy and population health (Mullin, 2010; Mund, 2011).

As the health care system became more complex, nursing leaders realized the need to provide nurses with sophisticated techniques to evaluate current policies and to develop innovative strategies for the future. The AACN's *Essentials of Master's Education in Nursing* (2011) recommended that APNs "advocate for policies that improve the health of the public and the profession of nursing." The AACN's *DNP Essentials* (2006) specified seven policy activities for the APN in Essential V, outlined at the beginning of this chapter. All of the Essentials addressed the expectation that APNs will assume the roles of leadership and advocacy in the health policy arena. Upon graduation APNs should have the knowledge and skills to advocate for effective, efficient, and equitable health care for individuals, groups, and populations.

The focus of advocacy depends not only on the APN's education but also on professional practice, personal experience, and motivation. A pediatric nurse practitioner observes that children in families who cannot afford insurance, but whose income is above a state-mandated threshold, do not qualify for government programs like Medicaid or for state health insurance programs. A psychiatric nurse practitioner discovers that a number of patients have been incarcerated instead of receiving appropriate treatment because psychiatric facilities in the area are overcrowded. A DNP graduate supervising a statewide tuberculosis program notices an increase in patient mortality. In each of the situations, the work environment may trigger an interest in a problem directly affected by health policies and laws. Regardless of clinical specialty, as members of the nursing profession, APNs have an interest in the on-going efforts to acquire an appropriate scope of practice and just reimbursement at the state and national levels (AACN, 2006; Mund, 2010).

Personal experience also plays a role in the choice of policies and issues most important to a nurse. A family member killed by a drunk driver, a spouse who lost health insurance after becoming unemployed, a child with a serious congenital disease may prompt an APN to assume an activist role with respect to those issues.

Motivation is arguably the strongest determinant of whether one will become an activist. An APN must want to bring about change through the political process. Political activism is time-consuming, often frustrating, and frequently confrontational. Successful advocates maintain a commitment to a goal that enables them to take the negative aspects of advocacy in stride.

Concern about a professional or personal experience may lead the APN to find out more about an issue through reading health care policy journals, accessing the Internet, attending professional meetings, or discussing the problem with a mentor (Mullin, 2010). As the APN learns more about a topic, the focus of advocacy sharpens. The APN may be further motivated to contact politicians and lawmakers to discuss their perspectives on the issue. If a policy or law is already in place, the APN examines it to determine if and how it can be improved.

"The goal of health policy ... is to contribute to improving the health of individuals and communities" (Aday et al., 2004). Even after a thorough assessment in which the effectiveness and efficiency of a policy have been established, the APN may be ambivalent about the direction advocacy should take because the perceived benefits to individual patients appear at odds with the perceived benefits to society (Mund, 2011). How does the APN decide on the most equitable course of action? Aday and her colleagues addressed this question using three paradigms that pertain to the just distribution of health care (Aday et al., 2004). The first paradigm is *distributive justice*. Adherents to this model have faith in individual autonomy and decision making. They believe that individuals are entitled to demand the health care that they need, regardless of the impact on the larger community. The second paradigm is *social justice*. Adherents to this model believe that society takes precedence over the individual. They believe that policies and laws should result in improved community health even though they result in a loss of benefits to an individual. The third paradigm, *deliberative justice*, takes a centrist position. Adherents to this model argue that through public discussion, policy makers can reach a compromise between individual rights and the general good. Although these paradigms are expressed in political discussions they have a philosophical foundation that reflects beliefs and values rather than facts. APNs will become more successful advocates if they understand their own and their opponents' philosophical perspectives on justice in health care policy.

There is another issue to consider before becoming politically active. A natural tension exists between advocacy and evaluation. In fact, there are evaluators who believe that supporting a specific policy or law threatens the essential open-mindedness and impartiality of the role (Fitzpatrick, Sanders, & Worthen, 2004). An APN who, as a result of education, experience, and motivation, chooses to become an activist should make an effort to maintain a certain detachment from the issues, to appreciate different viewpoints, and to reassess alternative options.

There are a number of approaches to political activism. One of the simplest is to join a professional organization (Hahn, 2009). There are numerous groups that provide support to nurses interested in advocacy. Professional organizations that are particularly relevant to the APN include American Association of Nurse Practitioners (AANP), the American Nurses Association (ANA), and the American Association of Colleges of Nursing (AACN). Organizations such as the American Association of Nurse Anesthetists (AANA) and the American College of Nurse Midwives (ACNM) provide a clinical focus. Professional organizations frequently have Political Action Committees (PACs) that offer a direct link to state and national legislators. These organization present opportunities for mentoring and facilitate collaboration with peers in developing successful strategies to evaluate and improve health care policy. Strategies may consist of meeting with legislators, preparing position statements and briefs, publishing in journals, giving interviews to the media, and organizing letter-writing campaigns (Betz, Smith, Melnyk, & Rickey, 2011; Mullin, 2010; Mund, 2011).

Some APNs may want to go a step further and assume a leadership role in advocacy. If that is the case, advanced education and experience are helpful. Universities, foundations, and professional associations offer advanced courses in leadership, health policy, and politics. Fellowships with agencies such as the Robert Wood Johnson Foundation provide a way to network with other health professionals who share common interests and to meet with policymakers at the local, state and, national levels (Mullin, 2010; Spross & Hanson, 2009). Ultimately, successful advocacy depends upon a long-term commitment of time, energy, and talent, a single-minded focus on an issue that is important to the APN, and an enthusiasm for the political process.

BOX 10.1 CASE STUDY: CHANGING POLICY WITH RESPECT TO TESTING FOR HIV

Phase 1

The first cases of what was later to be called the acquired immunodeficiency syndrome (AIDS) were reported in 1981. By 1984, the causative agent, human immunodeficiency virus (HIV), was discovered. Once the virus was known, it was possible to develop a test for antibodies to the virus. By 1985, very accurate tests were available that would determine if a person was HIV infected within a 6-month window after the infection occurred. By this time all of the routes of transmission had been identified—sexual, blood transfusion, needle sharing, mother-to-child transmission, and needle stick injuries to health care workers. Associating needle sharing with illicit drug use and male-to-male sexual behaviors with this infection led to stigmatizing of anyone who had the HIV infection.

Once the test was available, public health authorities recommended that persons who considered themselves at risk for infection obtain HIV testing. Some segments of the health care community advocated that all patients be tested to prevent transmission from patients to health care workers. The HIV activist community questioned the value of testing in that there was no treatment for the infection or for its sequelae. In addition, the policy was seen as a mechanism by which any male who sought testing could potentially be identified as being gay. Therefore, community activists opposed any testing that would identify those being tested. As result, the Centers for Disease Control and Prevention (CDC) issued guidelines that said that testing should be done only if the tested person was counseled about the meaning of the test before being tested and again when the result was reported. If the result was negative, post-test counseling also should include education on how to avoid future risk of becoming infected. If positive, counseling should include how to avoid transmission to others and when and where to seek medical care (CDC, 1986, 1987). The CDC funded testing sites where names would not be taken during the testing process. The CDC also recommended that all testing be voluntary and that there be readily accessible sites where the test could be done anonymously. Many states passed laws requiring the expressed consent of the patient for testing. The laws usually had provisions protecting the privacy of those who were found to be HIV infected. The exception to these guidelines and laws was screening for HIV of blood and tissue donations, which could be done without counseling or permission.

Questions for Phase 1

- How do the early CDC guidelines for testing fit the definition of a policy?
- How do the early testing guidelines fit the definition of a health policy?
- Are the guidelines an example of a public or a private health policy?

(*continued*)

- What was the context for the guidelines in terms of the science and technology?
- Who were the stakeholders during this first stage of testing?
- How did each group of stakeholders define the problem?
- What were the values and beliefs that determined the CDC's approach to testing?
- In what way were nurses stakeholders in implementing these new recommendations? _____

Phase 2

Eventually, epidemiologic and immunologic studies demonstrated that infection with HIV resulted in gradual destruction of the immune system, which typically occurred over 8 to 12 years. During most of this period, the infected person is asymptomatic. Toward the end of this asymptomatic period, infected adults may begin to experience opportunistic infections and cancers that meet the case definition for being classified as a case of AIDS. While AIDS was a reportable condition in all 50 states, HIV infection with patient names was not reportable in most states. This meant that tracking the growth and spread of the infection could only be done by analyzing AIDS cases, which reflected infections that had occurred 8 to 10 years earlier. Obviously, a much better system for tracking the epidemic would exist if persons with HIV infection but who had not progressed to AIDS would be reported to health departments.

Therefore, the CDC began encouraging state health departments to require reporting of HIV infections with patients' names. By 1988, 28 states required that HIV infections reported to the public health authorities include names. However, most of the states with large numbers of HIV-infected persons—including Florida, Texas, California, and New York—did not require reporting of HIV infection until 1999–2002. By 2003, 49 states and territories required such reporting. This slow accumulation of states requiring name-based reporting reflects the nature of the federal/state public health system in the United States. There is no national health authority that can require action by the states. Each state makes its own public health laws and regulations. The CDC can only provide evidence, suggest actions, and cajole state agencies to adopt its recommendations. In the case of name-based reporting, each state has had various levels of opposition and/or lethargy toward making HIV infection a reportable condition. In addition, requiring the reporting of HIV infection put an additional burden on state and local health departments. In most cases, additional funding was not made available to implement this new reporting requirement.

Questions for Phase 2

- What was the political and social context that determined whether states would require reporting of HIV infections by name?
- Who were the stakeholders in this situation?
- What optional policy alternatives might have been available to the CDC during the time period?
- In what way were nurses stakeholders in implementing these new recommendations?

Phase 3

With minor modifications, the 1986–1987 recommendations with regard to HIV infection were the main way of conducting HIV testing for the next several years. The science of HIV infection, however, continued to advance. In 1994, there was evidence that treating HIV-infected women with zidovudine (also known as AZT) during pregnancy and delivery, as well as treating their infants, would reduce the rate of mother-to-child transmission by two-thirds. This introduced the issue of whether testing should become mandatory or remain voluntary. The CDC recommended routine HIV counseling and voluntary testing of all pregnant women. Women were to be informed about the importance of being tested. The CDC recommended, however, that women should give permission to be tested (CDC, 1995). These recommendations were issued after a great deal of opposition against mandatory testing for HIV was expressed by activist groups.

By this time the CDC had conducted studies on the risk of transmission from an HIV-infected person to health care workers following needlestick injuries. They learned that there were approximately 3 transmissions per 1,000 needlestick injuries. The rate of transmission was lowered to one-seventh this rate (approximately 4 per 10,000) when the health care worker started a course of zidovudine within 24 hours of the needlestick. The rate of transmission became even lower if the health care worker took a course of the multidrug therapies that had become available.

Questions for Phase 3

- How did advances in science change how the problem for testing was defined?
- Who were the stakeholders during this phase?
- What were the alternatives to the screening policy for pregnant women?

(continued)

- What values seemed to underpin the policy to screen pregnant women?
- How did the data on outcomes influence policy for pregnant women and for health care workers?
- What kind of policy changes would be necessary for nurses working in inpatient obstetrical units to implement the CDC recommendations?
- What kind of policy changes would be necessary for nurses working in maternity clinics to implement the CDC recommendations?
- In what way were nurses stakeholders in implementing these new recommendations? _____

Phase 4

By the beginning of the 21st century, there were two major changes in HIV/AIDS. Highly effective drug therapies became available. These suppressed the level of the virus and allowed the immune system to reconstitute itself. This converted HIV infection from a death sentence to a manageable, chronic disease. In addition, much of the stigma associated with HIV infection had gone away. Individuals who had HIV infection were more likely to be considered as persons with a chronic disease than as deviants. This changed the focus of AIDS activists from concerns about testing to advocating for access to anti-HIV medications.

In 2001, the CDC issued new guidelines for HIV testing and counseling. These recommendations included most of the previous guidelines but emphasized interactive HIV counseling that was directed toward the patient's personal risk behaviors rather than generic, didactic risk reduction education. Several studies had shown that this form of education was more effective in promoting positive behavior changes. The CDC also recommended that health care providers screen their patients for risk in order to make HIV testing more efficient. These guidelines also raised the possibility that early identification of HIV infection and treatment with highly active antiretroviral treatment (HAART) could lead to reduced transmission of the virus (CDC, 2001). New scientific evidence had shown that HAART reduces the amount of circulating virus in blood, semen, and vaginal secretions. Experts believed that lower viral loads might result in lower rates of transmission.

Questions for Phase 4

- How did the definition of the problem of testing for HIV change during phase 4?

- Who are the stakeholders during this phase?
- What criteria (individual benefit vs. societal benefit) should be used to evaluate outcomes from the policy to screen and treat in order to prevent transmission?
- What organizational policies would be necessary to allow nurses to implement the one-on-one, tailored counseling that CDC was recommending?
- In what way were nurses stakeholders in implementing these new recommendations?

_____

Phase 5

In 2003, the CDC made several changes in its HIV testing guidelines following scientific advances and evaluations of the current HIV counseling and testing programs. In 2003, CDC-funded HIV test sites had provided approximately 2,000,000 tests and approximately 1% of these were newly discovered infections. However, of the newly discovered infections, 31% of those individuals did not receive their results. This was because the testing technology of that era required that confirmatory tests be done, which might take 1 to 2 weeks after blood was drawn before the test result was known and could be given to the individual. New tests using saliva had been developed that gave highly accurate results within 20 minutes. The test was relatively cheap, and no special equipment was required. Use of the test only required minimal training. Therefore, widespread use of this test was recommended for designated HIV testing sites and outreach programs to non-medical settings such as correctional facilities (CDC, 2003).

Additionally, the CDC found that many health care providers were unwilling or uneasy in doing risk assessment and pre-test counseling of their patients. Therefore, the CDC recommended that HIV testing be offered in settings serving populations with a high HIV prevalence. This could be done without ascertaining risk behaviors. These recommendations also removed the requirement for pre-test counseling (CDC, 2003).

Questions for Phase 5

- How did the definition of the problem for HIV testing change during phase 5?
- Who were the stakeholders during this phase?
- Besides the change in the science of testing, what other values were determining changes in the screening policies?

(continued)

- In what way were nurses stakeholders in implementing these new recommendations? _____

Phase 6

The CDC further revised and expanded its guidelines in 2006. The agency recommended that all persons between the ages of 13 and 64 be offered HIV testing at each encounter with a health care provider. This recommendation was based on the knowledge that approximately 25% of HIV-positive people did not know that they were infected and were continuing to transmit the virus to others. Other research determined that routinely offering testing was more likely to be acceptable to patients than providers interviewing them to ascertain if they had engaged in risky behaviors. Experts believed that routine testing would no longer stigmatize those who agreed to be tested. Another major change in these guidelines was a recommendation that pregnant women should be tested according to an "opt out" protocol. Instead of asking women if they would like to be tested, they would be told that they are going to be tested unless they refused. This change was based on research that showed that pregnant women would be more likely to consent to HIV testing if presented with an "opt out" choice (CDC, 2006).

The 2006 guidelines also emphasized that research now showed that patients with lower levels of circulating virus were less likely to transmit the virus. Reducing viral load was a major outcome of HAART so there was likely to be a prevention benefit if HIV infected individuals were identified at an earlier stage and began receiving treatment. There was also evidence that individuals who knew that they were HIV infected were less likely to put others at risk. There was also evidence that persons who did not know their HIV status were 3.5 times more likely to transmit the virus to others (CDC, 2006).

Questions for Phase 6

- How have program evaluation and outcome data influenced changes in screening policies during phase 6?
- Has there been a shift in how the benefits to society are weighed against the benefits to individuals?
- Who are the stakeholders during this phase?
- What are the expected outcomes from the policy changes during phase 6?
- What are your conclusions about the current screening policies?
- In what way were nurses stakeholders in implementing these new recommendations? _____

Questions for All Six Phases of the CDC Testing Recommendations

- Do you think that the CDC's organizational emphasis on prevention of disease was the driving factor during all six phases of their recommendations on testing?
- Do you think that nurses would have made different recommendations if they had been directing the policies on testing between 1986 and 2006? What would they be?

In 2011 there is emerging evidence that patients who are treated early in the infection—when their CD4 cells are still ≥500—are less likely to transmit the virus. It is likely that the CDC will establish a policy that will expand the screening criteria to detect and treat infected persons early.

You recognize that such testing will put a burden on your primary care practice and that of your colleagues. There is a window of opportunity here for you and other nurses to have input into either the development of the new policy or implementation of the policy.

- Who are the stakeholders now and what type of information do you want to provide to them?
- What additional information about the policy will you need to implement it?
- How would you evaluate whether the desired outcomes of the policy are met in your practice?

REFERENCES

Aday, L. U., Begley, C. E., Lairson, D. R., & Balkrishnan, R. (2004). *Evaluating the healthcare system: Effectiveness, efficiency, and equity*. Chicago, IL: Health Administration Press.

American Association of Colleges of Nursing. (2006). *The essentials of doctoral education for advanced practice nursing*. Retrieved from www.aacn.nche.edu

American Association of Colleges of Nursing. (2011). *The essentials of Master's education in nursing*. Retrieved from www.aacn.nche.edu

Betz, C. L., Smith, K. A., Melnyk, B. M., & Rickey, T. (2011). Disseminating evidence through publications, presentations, health policy briefs, and the media. In B. B. Melnyk & E. Fineout-Overholt (Eds.), *Evidence-based practice in nursing and healthcare* (2nd ed.). Philadelphia, PA: Wolters Kluwer/ Lippincott Williams & Wilkins.

Block, L. E. (2008). Health policy: What it is and how it works. In C. Harrington & C. L. Estes (Eds.), *Health policy: Crisis and reform in the U.S. health care delivery system* (5th ed., pp. 4–14). Sudbury, MA: Jones and Bartlett Publishers.

Centers for Disease Control and Prevention. (1986). Current trends: Additional recommendations to reduce sexual and drug abuse-related transmission of human T-lymphotropic virus type III/lymphadenopathy-associated virus. *Morbidity and Mortality Weekly Report, 35*(10), 152–155.

Centers for Disease Control and Prevention. (1987). Perspectives in disease prevention and health promotion public health service guidelines for counseling and antibody testing to prevent HIV infection and AIDS. *Morbidity and Mortality Weekly Report, 36*(31), 509–515.

Centers for Disease Control and Prevention. (1995). U.S. public health service recommendations for human immunodeficiency virus counseling and voluntary testing for pregnant women. *Morbidity and Mortality Weekly Report, 44*(RR-7), 1–15.

Centers for Disease Control and Prevention. (2001). Revised guidelines for HIV counseling, testing, and referral. *Morbidity and Mortality Weekly Report, 50*(RR-19), 1–58.

Centers for Disease Control and Prevention. (2003). Advancing HIV prevention: New strategies for a changing epidemic — United States 2003. *Morbidity and Mortality Weekly Report, 52*(15), 329–332.

Centers for Disease Control and Prevention. (2006). Revised recommendations for HIV testing of adults, adolescents, and pregnant women in health-care settings. *Morbidity and Mortality Weekly Report, 55*(RR-14).

Fitzpatrick, J. L., Sanders, J. R., & Worthen, B. R. (2004). *Program evaluation. Alternative approaches and practical guidelines.* Boston, MA: Pearson Education, Inc.

Hahn, J. (2009, August, September, October). Power dynamics, health policy, and politics. *Virginia Nurses Today.* Retrieved from www.VirginiaNurses.com

Hanley, B. E. (2002). Policy development and analysis. In D. J. Mason, J. K. Leavitt, & M. W. Chaffee (Eds.), *Policy and politics in nursing and health care* (pp. 55–69). St. Louis, MO: Saunders.

Longest, B. B. (2006). *Health policymaking in the United States* (4th ed.). Chicago, IL: Health Administration Press.

Mullin, M. H. (2010). DNP involvement in healthcare policy and advocacy. In L. A. Chism (Ed.), *The doctor of nursing practice: A guidebook for role development and professional issues* (pp. 141–167). Sudbury, MA: Jones and Bartlett Publishers.

Mund, A. (2011). Healthcare policy for advocacy in health care. In M. E. Zaccagnini & K. W. White (Eds.), *The doctor of nursing practice essential. A new model for advanced practice nursing* (pp.195–234). Sudbury, MA: Jones and Bartlett Publishers.

Spross, J. A., & Hanson, C. M. (2009). Clinical, professional, and systems leadership. In A. B. Hamric, J. A. Spross, & C. M. Hanson (Eds.), *Advanced practice nursing: An integrative approach.* St. Louis, MO: Saunders Elsevier.

Stokey, E., & Zeckhauser, R. (1978). *A primer for policy analysis.* New York, NY: W. W. Norton & Company Inc.

ELEVEN

Future Trends and Challenges in Evaluation

Christine A. Brosnan and Joanne V. Hickey

> *"We shall not cease from exploration*
> *And the end of all our exploring*
> *Will be to arrive where we started*
> *And know the place for the first time."*
>
> *T.S. Eliot*

INTRODUCTION

The previous chapters have addressed evaluation in health care from a number of different perspectives in which the APN will undoubtedly share now and in the future. There is no way to predict with any degree of certainty how events in the health care sector will pan out. Some developments seem more likely than others. However, there is, and will continue to be, an increased demand for comprehensive, high quality evaluation. The primary purpose of evaluation is to inform and support decision making based on relevant data that are collected, organized, and analyzed according to high standards of evaluation.

Although there are many approaches to evaluation, the type and design of an evaluation is linked to purpose. The complexity of health care delivery systems, organizations, and models of practice and care contribute to the complexity of decision making. Not only is complexity a hallmark of the current health care environment, but health care and all associated entities are undergoing extraordinary and unprecedented rapid changes that will add uncertainty to complexity. More fundamental and rapid changes are expected in the future as the United States' health enterprise struggles to align itself with the demands of a 21st century economy. The limited financial and human resources dedicated to health care, and the national imperative for quality and safety will continue to be major drivers for informed and responsible decision makers.

REFORMING HEALTH CARE

The Patient Protection and Affordable Care Act (P.L. 111–148) signed into law by President Barack Obama on March 23, 2010, addressed the challenge of providing quality health care for all Americans. The Affordable Care Act (ACA) was an attempt to overhaul the United States' health care system. The ACA provides for systematic and robust methods of evaluation in order to ensure more effective, efficient, and equitable health care. A few examples of some of the changes scheduled to occur over a period of 8 years are discussed in the following.

The ACA established the non-profit Patient Centered Outcomes Research Institute and charged it with evaluating the *effectiveness* of health care interventions and programs. The ACA authorized changes to Medicare that included linking payment to quality outcomes, using short-term and long-term indicators in measuring outcomes of care, and developing and evaluating home care programs to keep high risk patients out of hospitals. The law also directed the establishment of a national quality improvement strategy with the goal of improving the health care of individuals, groups, and populations (Anonymous, 2010).

There are a number of provisions in the Act aimed at improving health care *efficiency*. The ACA encouraged a shift from uneven and patchy health care to a comprehensive and accountable system. Through structural and process changes, the new health care system offers incentives to provide seamless and holistic health care (Ebner, 2010). An example is the provision for Accountable Care Organizations. These organizations will be composed of groups of health care professionals who collaborate in assessing patient needs, developing comprehensive and long-term plans of care, implementing the plans, and evaluating the effectiveness and efficiency of interventions and programs (Kocher & Sahni, 2010).

The ACA will result in increased access for about 32 million individuals who, prior to the law, could not afford care (Oberlander, 2010). The ACA accomplishes this through a combination of individual and employer insurance requirements and adjustments to public health programs. As a result, the vision of *equitable* health care in the United States becomes more realistic.

National legislation and public demand have raised the bar on what quality health care means. To meet the new standards, APNs and other health professions must provide health care that is effective, efficient, equitable, safe, patient-centered, and timely (Institute of Medicine, 2001). These attributes were derived from the Structure-Process-Outcome and the Effectiveness-Efficiency-Equity models. These models continue to offer clear blueprints for evaluating quality. However, there is consensus that methodological issues first identified by Donabedian and others persist and that they continue to challenge health care professionals in providing quality health care. Some of these issues are discussed in the following.

METHODOLOGICAL CHALLENGES TO IMPROVING HEALTH CARE QUALITY

It is essential that evaluation moves from using process indicators to predominantly using outcome indicators in measuring health care quality. Process indicators are a direct approach to evaluating whether health care is in compliance with best practice standards of a particular place and time. While they are helpful in measuring quality improvement in individual hospitals and agencies, they do not provide direct evidence about the effectiveness of care across geographical settings over time. Porter (2010) observed that the overwhelming majority of performance measures used by programs such as the Healthcare Effectiveness Data and Information Set (HEDIS) are still process indicators.

Selection of indicators is often influenced by the interests of those requesting an evaluation. Indicators that are essential to the health care marketplace and indicators that are essential to health care quality often differ. The marketplace is generally more interested in using process indicators and less interested in using the outcome indicators that are needed to objectively measure quality of care. For example, Lee noted that in his practice, clinic administrators routinely notified physicians about process indicators that were necessary for reimbursement such as the number of patient visits. They did not routinely notify physicians about outcome indicators that were necessary for evaluating effective care such as the number of patients seen in the emergency department (Lee, 2010). In comparing the differing perspectives on quality, Bowers and Kiefe (2002) observed that compared to health care evaluators, marketplace evaluators have a keen interest in measuring patient satisfaction with the hospital environment and amenities but are less inclined to measure risk adjustment or changes in health status.

Another challenge is identifying and adapting valid and reliable outcome indicators that can be standardized across settings. The implication of measures such as mortality rates that are frequently used by hospitals in establishing quality care can vary from setting to setting depending on the rigor of data collection and analysis. For example, evaluators in a certain location may fail to take into account patient risk factors or they may not reliably record data. The electronic health record (EHR) is seen as a way to address some of these issues but data input to EHRs also varies, and evaluating their usefulness in measuring quality has just begun. Provonost and Lilford (2011) cite the problems of missing data and the use of unclear and idiosyncratic algorithms in calculating outcomes as challenges to overcome.

A challenge that continues to puzzle evaluators is that, frequently, what is thought to be a link between short-term and long-term outcomes may not, in fact, exist. As an example, a 2006 study funded by the National Institutes of Health (NIH) involving 3,400 individuals sought to decrease heart attacks and strokes by using a combination therapy that included niacin, a medication thought to increase high density lipoproteins (HDL). The trial was scheduled to last 6 years but was stopped in May of 2011 (NIH, 2011). Researchers found that although niacin did increase HDL (a short-term outcome), it did not decrease the occurrence of heart attacks or strokes (a long-term outcome).

These challenges and others will not be easy to address but there has been progress in working toward accurately and precisely measuring health care quality. Because of their education and experience, APNs in collaboration with other health care professionals, can make a significant contribution to the endeavor. Suggestions for tackling the methodological issues that obstruct the systematic and objective evaluation of health care quality follow.

APNs should contribute to the development of standardized methods of measuring quality including nurse sensitive indicators. Currently, the number of nurse sensitive indicators is limited. The prevalence of pressure ulcers and frequency of falls are two measures that are frequently cited (Loan, Patrician, & McCarthy, 2011; Albanese et al., 2010). In developing methodologies, consideration should be given to the inclusion of short-term and long-term indicators, to valid and reliable data sources and data collection methods, and to transparent statistical analyses and algorithms used in calculating results. Outcomes should reflect the total patient experience and not just one intervention or the impact of one group of professionals (Provonost & Lilford, 2011; Porter, 2010).

APNs are in an ideal position to lead the quest for a culture of quality. Albanese et al. (2010) reported on a quality improvement and performance improvement program at the Hospital of the University of Pennsylvania that was based on Donabedian's model and supported by hospital leaders from nursing, medicine, and administration. The goal of the program was to establish a culture that encouraged nursing clinicians to become invested in continuous quality improvement efforts at the hospital. Structure and interdisciplinary input was provided by the hospital's quality improvement committee. Nurse clinicians collaborated to develop outcomes and performance measures derived from data. They created quality improvement standards that were applied and evaluated annually. Interdisciplinary dashboards enabled viewing of the current status of outcomes in each nursing specialty as well as their link to overall hospital goals. The initiative provided valuable patient data and succeeded in engaging staff nurses in continuing quality improvement activities.

The issues inherent in improving health care quality are daunting. Health care is complicated and change must occur at the micro, meso, and macro levels if it is to be successful. A program may be so large, complex, and fragmented that no one assumes responsibility for evaluation. State-mandated newborn screening is an example of such a program. It is interdisciplinary, multifaceted, and involves nursing care at the individual, group, and population level. The case study in Box 11.1 discusses some issues related to newborn screening quality and the role of the APN in addressing those issues.

BOX 11.1 STATE MANDATED NEWBORN SCREENING PROGRAMS

Newborn screening started when Dr. Robert Guthrie developed a test for phenylketonuria (PKU) in 1961. PKU is a rare genetic disorder that can result in mental retardation if a baby is not treated within a short time after birth. Babies who were screened and diagnosed with the disorder were given a modified diet that successfully prevented retardation. The benefit was clear, and over the years, PKU testing has helped thousands of children (Guthrie, 1992). Screening was strongly backed by politicians and consumer groups. Over time, other disorders were slowly added to the panel as testing became feasible. By the early 1990s, most states screened for about five or six conditions. And then, mass spectrometry was developed. This new method allowed technicians to screen for many more disorders using the same amount of blood as before. Today, a majority of the screening tests are analyzed by mass spectrometry. States are now able to screen for over 60 conditions (National Newborn Screening and Genetics Resource Center, 2010).

Newborn screening is mandated by every state and the District of Columbia and, as a result, approximately 4 million children are screened annually. But other than that mandate, screening varies widely among the states. In Vermont and Minnesota parents may refuse screening for any reason, while in Texas parents can only refuse on religious grounds. In many states they cannot refuse. Maryland asks parents to sign a consent form before screening. Some states require that each newborn have one complete screening panel, some require two, and others require one panel but recommend a second especially if the first screen is done on the first day of life. The number of tests in a screening panel also varies widely, with some states choosing to provide about 30 tests and others choosing to provide twice that amount. Each state decides how to finance its own screening program and how much it will charge (National Newborn

(continued)

Screening and Genetics Resource Center, 2010). Recently, there has been controversy around the issue of destroying or keeping the filter paper used in the collection of the blood specimen. (The President's Council on Bioethics, 2008; Rothwell et al., 2011).

Although wide variation exists among the states there is agreement that states need to follow general guidelines in administering screening programs including education, proper testing, follow-up, diagnosis, and evaluation (The President's Council on Bioethics, 2008). There is consensus that parents should be informed about what disorders are involved, how the tests will be done, what they should do if the tests are positive, and where they can go for follow-up and treatment. Everyone agrees that there should be an established process for pricking the infant's heel to collect the blood, for placing the blood on filter paper, and for sending the filter paper to a laboratory for analysis. There should be a plan for analyzing the blood and for establishing the cut-off point that separates a positive from a negative result. There should be guidelines about where to send the results if the test is positive and who will be responsible for making sure that parents know where to take their baby for follow-up. If a baby is diagnosed with a disorder there should be an effective treatment. Finally, all states should have a way of evaluating programs.

Nursing has an essential and continuing role in newborn screening. In the hospital, nurses provide information about the program to new parents and are usually designated to collect the blood specimen. Nurses are often the coordinators of the State Health Department Newborn Screening Programs. As coordinators they respond to questions from families and act as liaisons between the health department and other health professionals. Nurses frequently provide and coordinate care in the pediatric clinics to which the results are reported. Public health nurses may make home visits to determine why parents have not responded to notification about an abnormal screen. Finally, nurses collaborate with other health care professionals in providing long-term care to children diagnosed with a disorder.

Evaluating a complex and fragmented program like newborn screening may be overwhelming, but at each point of patient contact, nurses have an opportunity and a responsibility to become involved in evaluation activities. Examples of evaluation activities are described in the following.

1. An APN coordinating maternal-child units in a large hospital assumes responsibility for evaluating the literacy level, clarity, and language of the educational materials provided to parents. The APN analyzes how much time is spent with parents discussing the programs and the parents' understanding of what is being done. An evaluation reveals that most parents do not

understand the newborn screening process because of language and literacy barriers. The APN coordinates a team that develops new bilingual educational materials that are aimed at a ninth grade reading level.

2. An APN practicing in a pediatric clinic observes that there is a lack of coordination in notifying parents about positive screening tests and in ensuring that parents comply with follow-up recommendations. The APN joins other clinicians in establishing clinic protocol that standardizes notification and follow-up. Process and outcome indicators are monitored regularly.

3. An APN employed by a state health department as Coordinator of newborn screening activities observes that one of the tests has a large number of false positive results. The APN collaborates with members of the newborn screening team including physicians and laboratory technicians to evaluate the abnormal cut-off value of the screening test. The team analyzes the impact that changing the cut-off value will have on the frequency of false positive and false negative results. The team submits a report of their recommendations to designated administrators of the health department and clinical specialists in the state.

4. An APN whose clinical practice involves newborn screening regularly attends national meetings on the subject. The APN volunteers to serve on a national committee studying the storage and use of residual blood on filter paper.

Collaborating with nurses and other health care professionals in evaluating the quality of each patient contact in a large and complex program like newborn screening not only improves quality of health care but expands nursing's influence in developing programs and policies. Are there other examples of evaluation activities that should engage the APN?

The challenges for thoughtful and systematic evaluations that can inform decision making have never been greater. A crossroad has been reached in that an evaluation plan will be required before approval of funding of any project is initiated. In addition, a substantive evaluation will be required at the completion of any project to determine outcomes and value added. Health care providers have been forced to recognize that health care is a business, and as such, clinicians must be cognizant of a business model that includes evaluation of return on investment. This transition from a mindset of endless available resources to one of limited resources that must be wisely used and justified has shifted how health professionals must think. Making a decision is choosing one option over other options including recognizing intended and unintended consequences. It is comprehensive, valid, and reliable information from well-conceived and conducted evaluations that assists decision makers in making the best choices.

Many decisions are "high stake" decisions that will have a significant impact on how and what kind of health care and health policies are implemented. Quality indicators for evaluations include comprehensiveness, contextual relevancy, focus on the information needs of the user, validity, reliability, transparency, balanced information (e.g., control of bias), and fairness. Because of the demand for evaluation of the relative effectiveness of the various diagnostics, procedures, devices, pharmaceuticals, guidelines, protocols, and other interventions in clinical practice, the APN will be invited to participate in evaluation both as a leader and team member.

SCOPE OF EVALUATION EXPECTATIONS AND APNs

APNs are considered by the nursing profession, other professions, and society to be clinical experts by virtue of their education and experience. The expectation of evaluation has been included in graduate education at the master's level in nursing, but it has generally been underplayed and defined within the context of the individual patient for achieving very specific outcomes. The emerging and growing cadre of graduates of doctor of nursing practice programs increases the expectation of clinical scholars who have a deep and substantive knowledge of evaluation and who can lead evaluation efforts to inform the transformation of the health care system. The scope and depth of evaluation is one area of professional differentiation of performance within master's and doctoral nursing education and competency.

The following highlights major areas for evaluation competencies in which APNs are needed.

Standards, Guidelines, and Protocols

APNs must be able to evaluate standards, guidelines, and protocols. As discussed in Chapter 7, standards are broad statements that address expectations for professional performance and care. The APN must understand applicable standards in order to be able to evaluate current standards of performance and care for relevance to contemporary practice. Within the context of evidence-based guidelines and protocols, a major responsibility of APNs is to evaluate guidelines and protocols to be sure that they are aligned with current and valid evidence of best practices. Keeping up with the published scientific literature and evaluating current practices for needed update are huge and ongoing commitments that are directly linked to quality patient outcomes. It is an expectation that APNs will be leaders in this realm of clinical practice.

Models of Practice and Care

Another important responsibility of the APN is to evaluate models of practice and care based on best practices and an understanding of the local contextual environment in which practice occurs and care is delivered. For example, concurrent with the responsibility for providing the best care shown to lead to the best patient outcomes, the APN must evaluate the currently used models of practice and care to determined gaps and unmet needs. Much discussion centers around transitional care and niche care for selected populations, which could lead to better, more convenient, and cost-effective care. As patients move along the continuum of care, many gaps are evident. By most accounts, fragmentation of care is common, and it needs to be replaced by seamless integrated systems. For example, in an obstetrical unit in a major facility, an APN noted that mothers and babies were not being discharged on weekends because there was no staff available to conduct newborn screening examinations. This tied up beds for an extra two days and was inconvenient for patients and families. There was also a substantial economic loss to the facility that was not reimbursable by insurers. By initiating a pediatric nurse practitioner weekend clinic, bed flow, cost, and convenience were addressed. The clinic did not just happen. It took an astute APN to recognize the problem, conduct a comprehensive evaluation, propose options with risk-benefit analyses, prepare a business plan, and employ leadership skills to move an innovative solution through the organization and decision makers.

Another example of evaluation is appraising a current facility's readiness for a major shift in focus, such as to a patient-family centered model of care. What would it take for an organization to make the cultural change from its current model of a patient being directed by an interdisciplinary team to a patient-family centered model? A comprehensive evaluation would be needed to address the multiple and interrelated structural and processes-driven changes that would need to be address in order to make the transition.

All quality care is interdisciplinary; it takes a village of health professionals representing a number of disciplines to provide comprehensive care that leads to optimal outcomes. The APN has a huge role in evaluating teams for effectiveness. As discussed in Chapter 9, interdisciplinary collaborative teams are the fundamental pivotal hubs of care. High performance teams are dynamic and highly interactive groups of professionals focused on mutually accepted goals. Team communications are very complex and are subject to misunderstandings and disruption. APNs, as both members of interdisciplinary teams and as outside evaluators, can contribute to ongoing optimal group function.

Acquisitions

Employers expect APNs to participate in the decision making surrounding acquisition of new equipment and other resources to support health care delivery. These purchases often represent major expenditures and capital investments. The APN must be able to determine how the item will impact care delivery and concurrent changes in practice, current equipment and workflow, patient outcomes, care provider user-friendliness (e.g., ease of use, reliability, workflow), and patient acceptance (e.g., comfort, acceptability), and to assess its potential for reimbursement, and cost. As a member of a team providing input on acquisitions, the input of the APN must be based on a systematic and thorough evaluation of current resources and comparison to the proposed products to determine feasibility and usefulness to the practice setting. APNs understand the spectrum of questions that emerge throughout the product or intervention lifecycle in clinical practice and can therefore ask pertinent questions that contribute to an evaluation. The emerging science of comparative effectiveness should assist the APN in providing data-driven input related to acquisitions.

For example, the digital revolution is reconfiguring practice and care in health care facilities. Multi-million dollar contracts for digital information systems are major capital investments that require a comprehensive evaluation of clinical and organizational practice patterns for interface with current databases and systems. Many organizations have found, to their dismay, that their current information systems do not interface with the newly purchased system. Although most APNs do not have the technical knowledge to question how the interface might occur, they do have the expertise to raise questions from the clinician perspective. Do new orders for drugs entered into the electronic order sheet go electronically to the pharmacy, or do the orders have to been reentered into a separate pharmacy order system? Can arrangements be made to mine data from large databases so that the unit has a monthly report on admissions, lengths of stay, infections, and other items of interest for quality improvement purposes? Chapter 6 has addressed APNs and evaluation of health care information systems and patient technology.

Current Programs and Program Development

Evaluation of current and potential programs is often linked to practice-care issues and health policy. Programs are organized services that address the needs of a designated population of patients. APNs are often requested to conduct a program evaluation. The impetus for a program evaluation might be to determine comprehensive outcomes of a program (e.g., patient outcomes, satisfaction, and cost) and possible interest in expanding, revising, or deleting a program. Of all of the focus areas of evaluation, program evaluation is the most frequently addressed. Numerous books, articles, and websites readily offer information on program evaluation. The APN should be familiar with these resources. An evaluation to establish the need for a new parent education program about newborn screening is an example of one type of evaluation that the APN may conduct. Another example might be to evaluate a current program to confirm the need for expansion. A current heart failure program may be evaluated to determine if a special program should be established for women with heart failure to address their special needs. There are endless opportunities for APNs to engage in program evaluation.

Health Policy

One recommendation in *The Future of Nursing: Leading Change, Advancing Health* (Institute of Medicine, 2011) is that nurses should become full partners with physicians and other health professionals to redesign health care in the United States. The greatest opportunity for this recommendation to be fulfilled is in the health policy arena. Health policy is where the rules and regulations that control practice and care issues are influenced and negotiated. The more than three million professional nurses in the United States nurses represent the largest health care workforce compared to other health care professionals. Their voices need to be heard at the health policy table at the local, state, and national levels. It is often the APN who is the voice for nurses and who speaks as advocates for patients and quality care. APNs must understand the processes involved in influencing health policy and develop the competencies to participate in the process. Several chapters in this book including Chapters 3, 5, 8, and 10 address this critical leadership role. In order to be an effective participant, the APN must be able to evaluate current and proposed health policies.

For example, at the local level a current organizational policy on scheduling of new patients may be creating a hardship for some patients. Perhaps in approving this policy there was no thought about the impact on patients. The APN could assume the advocacy role for the patient. An example of health policy on the state level is the requirement for frequent physician oversight of nurse practitioners in a rural underserved area. If the closest physicians are 75 miles away from the clinic and unable to travel that distance every few weeks to review charts, the nurse practitioner may be unable to practice and patients may be left without any health care. On the national level APNs are often invited to serve on committees and boards that make recommendations about health policy. APN participation is critical to providing the advocacy voice for patients and quality care.

Peer and Self Evaluation

Finally, evaluation of self and peers to determine performance and to develop an individualized development plan is a professional responsibility. The American Nurses Association (2010) has outlined both the expectation and process for peer and self-evaluation as tools for professional growth and development to support high quality patient care and outcomes.

DEVELOPING AND MAINTAINING COMPETENCY IN EVALUATION

The increased expectation and future role for APNs to be experts in evaluation raises the question of how to develop and maintain evaluation expertise. APNs need to recognize their important and expanding role in evaluation and to embrace it. An evaluation provides an opportunity to inform and influence data-driven decision making that is based on a systematic process. The following lists recommendations for the APN to develop and maintain expertise in evaluation:

- Learn all you can about evaluation through academic course work, continuing education programs, and reading.
- Work with others who have expertise in evaluation for mentoring experiences.
- Conduct your own competency analysis and achievement of objectives; set a timeline and review and update periodically.
- Include evaluation as a focus in your individualized development plan and monitor your progress.

In the future, with the higher expectation of evaluation expertise for APNs, job retention and promotion will be tied, in part, to expertise in evaluation. Therefore, career planning should include attention to competency development and maintenance in the many forms of evaluation.

Selected online resources to help APNs expand their knowledge of evaluation are listed in the following.

Online Resources

Agency for Healthcare Research and Quality (http://www.ahrq.gov/)
A federal agency that provides funding, clinical information, and guidelines for
    health care quality.
American Evaluation Association (http://www.eval.org)
An international professional organization that offers literature, courses, and meet-
    ings focused on program and other types of evaluation.
Center for Health Care Evaluation (http://www.chce.research.va.gov/)
Part of the United States Department of Veteran Affairs, CHCE provides information
    to improve health care quality for veterans and the entire population.
The Commonwealth Fund (http://www.commonwealthfund.org/)
Provides information on health care reform, health system performance measures,
    and health care quality including state report cards.

Institute for Healthcare Improvement (http://www.ihi.org/ihi)
Provides information on increasing effectiveness and efficiency in the health care system, and describes key indicators and protocols for bringing about change.
National Quality Forum (http://www.qualityforum.org/Home.aspx)
Offers instruction on measuring health care quality including the use of dashboards to present evaluation results.
Robert Wood Johnson Foundation. (2004). (http://www.rwjf.org/pr/product. jsp?cd=18657)
A guide to evaluation primers. Provides a critique of the strengths and weaknesses of 11 frequently cited primers on evaluation.
W. K. Kellogg Foundation (http://www.wkkf.org)
Supports evaluation activities and tools including providing an evaluation handbook.

REFERENCES

Albanese, M. P., Evans, D. A., Schantz, C. A., Bowen, M., Piesieski, P., & Polomano, R. C. (2010). Engaging clinical nurses in quality and performance improvement activities. *Nursing Administration Quarterly, 34*(3), 226–245.

American Nurses Association. (2010). *Scope and standards of practice* (2nd ed.). Silver Spring, MD: Author.

Anonymous. (2010). *Focus on health reform. Summary of new health reform law* (Publication #8061). Kaiser Family Foundation. Retrieved from www.kff.org

Bowers, M. R., & Kiefe, C. I. (2002). Measuring health care quality: Comparing and contrasting the medical and the marketing approaches. *American Journal of Medical Quality, 17*(4), 136–144.

Ebner, A. L. (2010). What nurses need to know about health care reform. *Nursing Economics, 28*(3), 191–194.

Guthrie, R. (1992). The origin of newborn screening. *Screening, 1*, 5–15.

Institute of Medicine. (2001). *Crossing the quality chasm: A new health system for the 21st century.* Washington, DC: National Academies Press.

Institute of Medicine. (2011). *The future of nursing: Leading change, advancing health.* Washington, DC: The National Academies Press.

Kocher, R., & Sahni, N. R. (2010). Physicians versus hospitals as leaders of accountable care organizations. *New England Journal of Medicine, 363*(27), 2579–2582.

Lee, T. H. (2010). Putting the value framework to work. *New England Journal of Medicine, 363*(26), 2481–2483.

Loan, L. A., Patrician, P. A., & McCarthy, M. (2011). Participation in a national nursing outcomes database: Monitoring outcomes over time. *Nursing Administration Quarterly, 35*(1), 72–81.

National Institutes of Health. (2011, May 26). *The national heart, lung, and blood institutes.* Retrieved from http://public.nhlbi.nih.gov/newsroom/home/GetPressRelease. aspx?id=2792

National Newborn Screening and Genetics Resource Center. (2010, January). Retrieved from http://genes-r-us.uthscsa.edu/

Oberlander, J. (2010). Beyond repeal-the future of health care reform. *New England Journal of Medicine, 363*(24), 2277–2279.

Porter, M. E. (2010). What is value in health care? *New England Journal of Medicine,* *363*(26), 2477–2481.

Provonost, P. J., & Lilford, R. (2011). A road map for improving the performance of performance measures. *Health Affairs, 30*(4), 569–573.

Rothwell, E. W., Anderson, R. A., Burbank, M. J., Goldenberg, A. J., Lewis, M. H., Stark, L., … Botkin, J. R. (2010). Concerns of newborn blood screening advisory committee members regarding storage and use of residual newborn screening blood spots. *American Journal of Public Health, 101*(11), 2111–2116.

The President's Council on Bioethics. (2008). *The changing moral focus of newborn screening: An ethical analysis by the President's Council on Bioethics.* Washington DC.

Index